The Pink Salt Trick Recipe for Fast Weight Loss

Your Simple, Natural Morning Ritual to Boost Metabolism, Control Cravings, and Burn Fat – All Without Strict Diets or Expensive Supplements!

Avery Quinn

© Copyright 2025 – Avery Quinn

All rights reserved.

The content contained within this book may not be reproduced, duplicated, or transmitted without direct written permission from the author or the publisher.

Under no circumstances will any blame or legal responsibility be held against the publisher or author for any damages, reparation, or monetary loss due to the information contained within this book, either directly or indirectly.

Legal Notice:

This book is copyright-protected. It is only for personal use. You cannot amend, distribute, sell, use, quote, or paraphrase any part of this book's content without the author's or publisher's consent.

Disclaimer Notice:

Please note that the information contained within this document is for educational purposes only. All efforts have been made to present accurate, up-to-date, reliable, and complete information. No warranties of any kind are declared or implied. Readers acknowledge that the author does not render legal, financial, medical, or professional advice. The content within this book has been derived from various sources. Please consult a licensed professional before attempting any techniques outlined in this book.

By reading this document, the reader agrees that under no circumstances is the author responsible for any direct or indirect losses incurred as a result of the use of the information contained within this document, including, but not limited to, errors, omissions, or inaccuracies.

Table of Contents

Introduction 5

Chapter 1: The Origins of Himalayan Pink Salt 9
    What Is Himalayan Pink Salt 10

Chapter 2: Facts and Myths About Pink Salt 15
    Common Myths 15
    Risks and Cautions 18

Chapter 3: Core Recipes Using Pink Salt 19
    Recipe Variations 20
    Traditional Drinks 29
    Tips for Success 36

Chapter 4: Pink Daily Recipes 38
    Snacks for Craving Control 38
    Anti-Inflammatory On-the-Go Foods 44
    Pink Salt Smoothies 50
    On-the-Go Tips 56

Chapter 5: Morning Rituals and Holistic Well-Being Using the Pink Salt Trick 58
    Morning Pink Salt Rituals 59
    Evening Salt Routines 61
    Gentle Evening Movement Synergy 62
    Mindfulness Practices 63
    Calming Yoga Flows to Enhance Mineral Absorption 64

Chapter 6: 7-Day Pink Salt Trick Healing Challenge 66
    How the Challenge Works 66
    7-Day Plan 68
    Tracking Progress 71

Chapter 7: Weight Loss Management After the Challenge 74
    Sustaining the Pink Salt Trick 75
    Overcoming Challenges 79

Chapter 8: The Pink Salt Trick for Lasting Well-Being 80
    Beauty with Pink Salt 80

    Illness Recovery...83
    Holistic Practices with Pink Salt..86
    Face Yoga and Pink Salt Facial Mist..86
    Scalp Massage + Pink Salt Scalp Scrub...87
    Reflexology + Pink Salt Foot Soak..88
    Tongue Scraping + Pink Salt Mouth Rinse..90
    Acupressure + Pink Salt Compress..91
    Dry Brushing + Gua Sha with Pink Salt...93
    Bringing it Together..94

Conclusion...96

References..99

Introduction

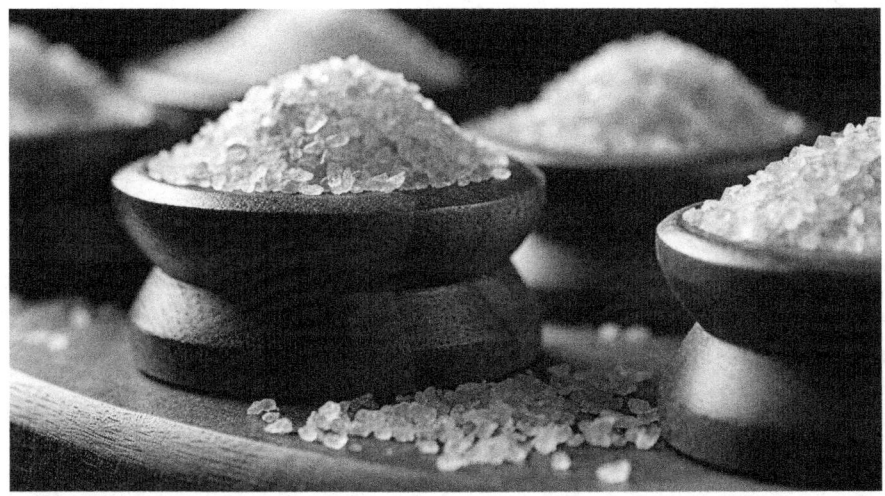

HAVE YOU EVER spotted something online that seemed way too easy to actually work? That was exactly my reaction when I first saw the buzz about the pink salt trick for melting away stubborn pounds. Pink salt? The pretty stuff on fancy restaurant tables? Turns out, this unassuming crystal might just be your metabolism's new best friend.

Let's get real for a second, losing weight today is a total minefield. One minute you're cutting carbs, the next you're doing burpees until you collapse, and somehow your jeans still feel just as tight! Why? Because most methods completely miss what's actually happening inside your body. When your metabolism is crawling, hormones are haywire, and your gut is on fire, counting calories is like using a squirt gun to fight a forest fire.

Here is the uncomfortable truth: millions of women (especially those of us over 35) are secretly fighting invisible weight blockers that no gym membership can fix. Our bodies are screaming for help. We're dehydrated, nutrient-starved, and completely unable to burn fat. The result? Exhaustion by 3 PM, bloat that makes you look 5 months pregnant by dinner, and chocolate cravings that hit like a freight train when your boss sends you "that email."

As we move into our 30s, our bodies start seriously slacking on hormone production. Suddenly, you're dealing with:

- Stubborn muffin tops may appear out of nowhere.
- "Wait, what was I saying?" moments mid-conversation.
- A digestive system that seems perpetually annoyed with you.
- Mood swings that make you question your sanity.

These aren't annoying inconveniences. They're flashing warning signs of metabolic chaos paired with hormonal rebellion. And our modern food-like products, non-stop stress, and nutrient-bankrupt habits are throwing gasoline on this metabolic dumpster fire.

The good news is that there is a ridiculously simple, science-backed reset button hiding in your kitchen!

Imagine jumpstarting your body's fat-burning engine without downing sketchy stimulants, enduring miserable cleanses, or saying goodbye to foods you actually enjoy. That's exactly what *The Pink Salt Trick* delivers: a super simple daily ritual using mineral-packed Himalayan salt that floods your cells with exactly what they need while switching on your body's forgotten fat-melting pathways.

The Pink Salt Trick has been written to help you understand the approach that has been making waves in 2025. We uncover exactly how it transforms your biology, and why coupling the pink salt method with other easy-to-follow techniques can finally be the breakthrough moment your struggling body deserves.

At its heart, the Pink Salt Trick is a deliciously simple hydration ritual that harnesses the power of authentic Himalayan pink salt mixed with pure water. Don't be fooled by its simplicity, this ancient wellness practice delivers a powerful metabolic reboot by supporting deep hydration, restoring crucial minerals, and revitalizing your digestive system.

This extraordinary salt contains over 19 trace minerals and electrolytes your body craves, magnesium, potassium, calcium, iron, and more, elements that balance your pH, regulate your fluid levels, and fire up the enzymes that kickstart your fat-burning furnace.

Recent research has finally caught up to what traditional healers have known forever: mineral balance is a game-changer. Regular intake of natural electrolytes has been proven to:

- Skyrocket your energy levels while hydrating your cells from the inside out
- Rev up metabolic function and accelerate fat breakdown
- Support optimal thyroid performance and hormone balance
- Crush those maddening sugar cravings and emotional eating triggers

Why This Book

Get ready for your total body transformation! I've packed these pages with everything you need to revolutionize not just how you look, but how you feel from the inside out. No more half-measures or temporary fixes. This is about reclaiming your metabolic power for good.

In the chapters to come, you'll discover recipes that work with your hormones instead of against them. But that's just the appetizer! I'm challenging you to a 7-day metabolic reset that will change everything you thought you knew about your body. This isn't some miserable starvation week, it's seven days of strategic eating, drinking, and moving that flushes out metabolic roadblocks and switches your body back to fat-burning mode.

And because I know weight loss is about more than the scale, I've loaded this guide with game-changing beauty and recovery hacks. Learn how the same minerals that torch belly fat can transform your skin, hair, and energy levels. These tips aren't just about looking good in your jeans (though you absolutely will), they're about rebooting your entire system for all-day energy that doesn't crash and burn.

I'm here to let you know that your body is not broken! It's just mineral-starved and desperate for the right kind of attention. And I'm about to show you exactly how to give it what it needs to thrive. Now is the time to take back your health, boost your metabolism, and lose weight fast!

Bonus Page

Are you loving your results with the Pink Salt Trick? Are you ready to pair your Pink Salt Trick with something even **more** powerful?

I couldn't possibly include this controversial weight loss secret in the main book (it's **that** powerful), but as a valued reader, you deserve access to **every** tool in my transformation arsenal!

The Brazilian Mounjaro drink combines a powerful ingredient with a unique preparation method that:

- Accelerates fat-burning by up to 3X compared to pink salt alone.
- Targets the most stubborn belly and thigh fat that won't budge.
- Reduces hunger signals while **boosting** energy levels.
- Works while you sleep to maximize overnight fat metabolism

When paired with your Pink Salt Trick, the results can be absolutely extraordinary!

Claim your free gift now by scanning the QR code below to download your **free** Brazilian Mounjaro guide instantly!

Chapter 1:
The Origins of Himalayan Pink Salt

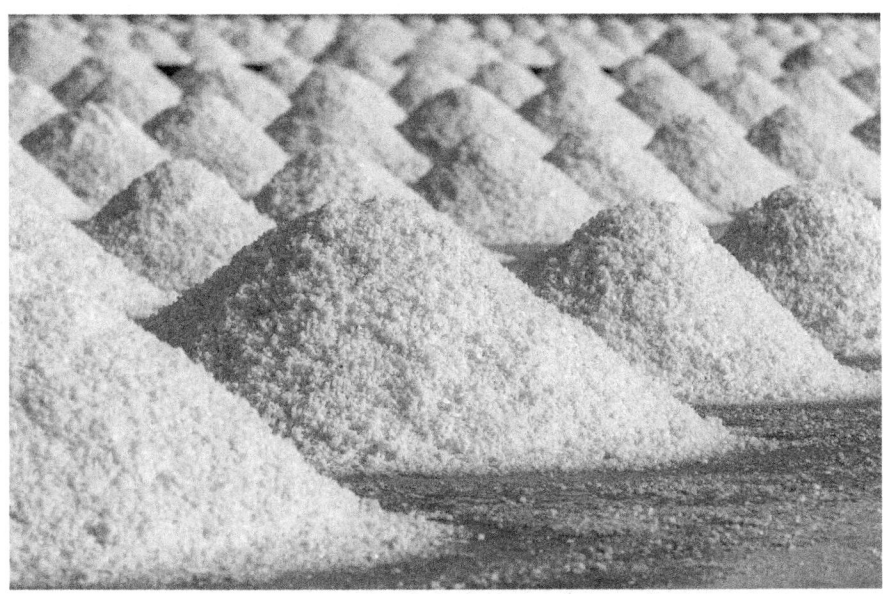

PINK SALT SEEMS to have hit our grocery shelves as if it came out of nowhere. Before we knew it, the pretty pink granules took over, costing three times more than regular table salt, despite "health pundits" trying to convince us it was nothing more than table salt.

Its resurgence may have been swift, but Himalayan pink salt has been quietly transforming health practices for centuries before it ever hit your local grocery store shelf.

While modern wellness trends come and go faster than celebrity relationships, this rose-colored crystal has staying power for good reason. Formed over 250 million years ago when ancient oceans evaporated and left mineral-rich deposits in what's now Pakistan's Punjab region, Himalayan pink salt is literally fossilized history packed with health secrets our ancestors understood intuitively.

Traditional Ayurvedic healers weren't messing around when they prescribed salt therapy for everything from respiratory issues to digestion problems. They recognized what modern science is finally catching up to: the mineral composition in this unprocessed salt speaks your body's language in ways that processed table salt simply cannot.

What Is Himalayan Pink Salt

Despite the controversy, the pretty crystals in your clear salt grinder are not the same as table salt. Himalayan pink salt comes from the ancient Khewra Salt Mine in Pakistan's Punjab region, part of the Salt Range formation that's been harvesting nature's mineral treasure for over 2,000 years. These salt deposits formed when primordial oceans evaporated millions of years ago, leaving behind concentrated minerals locked in time.

What makes this salt drop-dead gorgeous isn't just for show. The distinctive blush pink to deep rose coloring comes from its iron oxide content. But the real magic isn't just what gives it that social media-worthy hue. While processed table salt is just sodium chloride stripped of everything useful (then loaded with anti-caking agents you can't pronounce), Himalayan pink salt contains up to 84 trace minerals and elements! So why do gurus insist that pink salt and mineral salt are the same thing?

The difference is in the name. Mineral salt and Pink salt are one and the same. Both contain trace minerals and elements. Table salt is not the same. It is refined through an arduous chemical transformation to strip away these trace minerals to leave it pure white and pure sodium, paired with an anti-caking agent and added iodine.

This means unless you are adding **mineral** salt to your diet, your body is screaming for magnesium, potassium, calcium, zinc, and dozens more that play crucial roles in everything from nerve function to muscle control.

Think about it: these are the same minerals that expensive supplements promise to deliver, yet here they are in this unassuming crystal that costs pennies per serving while you're splashing hundreds of dollars a month on supplements!

When your cells are starving for these trace elements (and trust me, if you're eating the Standard American Diet, they absolutely are), your body's metabolic processes start misfiring like an engine running on fumes. Your thyroid slows down, your digestion gets sluggish, and suddenly those stubborn fat deposits seem impossible to budge.

What's truly mind-blowing is that this salt contains less sodium per teaspoon than table salt. Before you come at me, yes, all salts contain about 98% sodium, but pink salt's crystal size means that you receive less of the good stuff and more of the minerals your body needs.

When you understand how these microscopic mineral particles interact with your body's systems, suddenly it makes perfect sense why something as simple as switching your salt could create such dramatic changes. And we're just scratching the surface of what this ancient pink powerhouse can do for your metabolism!

Traditional Uses

Long before pink salt became the darling of social media food photographers, it was revered across ancient healing traditions for its powerful effects on the body.

In Ayurvedic medicine, a 5,000-year-old healing system that somehow knew more about our bodies than modern science is just now discovering, pink salt was called "saindhava lavana" and considered the king of salts. Ayurvedic texts specifically singled it out as the salt that alleviates the imbalanced bio-energies and was one of the few substances recommended for daily consumption.

Traditional healers didn't have fancy laboratories, but they weren't stupid. They observed what happened when people used different substances and kept detailed records for centuries. What they discovered about pink salt was that it had unique properties for:

- Supercharging digestion and preventing that embarrassing post-meal bloating.
- Pulling toxins out of the body (hello, natural detox that doesn't require drinking nasty green juice!).
- Balancing internal fluids to prevent swelling and water retention.
- Energizing the body when fatigue hits (without the crash that comes from those sugary energy drinks).

But it wasn't just Ayurvedic medicine. Ancient Greeks used pink salt to clear airways and improve breathing. Throughout parts of Asia, salt therapy has been used for respiratory conditions for generations. People would visit natural salt caves to breathe in the mineral-rich air, a practice that modern "salt rooms" in fancy spas are now charging top dollar to recreate. Our ancestors knew that inhaling those tiny salt particles could help open airways, reduce inflammation, and clear out lung gunk—all without a single pharmaceutical side effect!

But perhaps the most overlooked traditional use is hydration and energy balance. When consumed in water, traditional healers observed that pink salt helped "regulate the water content throughout your body" and promoted "the generation of hydroelectric energy in body cells." In plain English, it helped people stay properly hydrated (not just water-logged) and maintained their energy levels without stimulants.

Think about how revolutionary this is! While modern sports drinks are loaded up with artificial colors, flavors, and questionable ingredients to "replace electrolytes," traditional cultures were simply adding a pinch of mineral-rich salt to water and experiencing the same benefits naturally.

Modern Resurgence

From ancient wisdom to modern obsession, pink salt is having a major moment! Remember when it was just sitting quietly in some health food store corner? Now it's everywhere from high-end kitchens to wellness influencer feeds to those lit-up salt lamps that suddenly appeared in everyone's living room overnight!

What sparked this crystal comeback? It all started with wellness tastemakers who turned this humble mineral into the crown jewel of the clean eating movement. When the rich and famous started gushing about their pink salt rituals, the rest of us mere mortals couldn't help but wonder if we were missing out on some ancient secret to looking and feeling amazing.

The timing couldn't have been better. Just as people were getting sick of processed everything, here comes this gorgeous, rose-colored crystal promising to be the antidote to our modern, chemical-filled existence. It looked different, tasted different, and had a whole backstory about ancient oceans and Himalayan mountains that made sprinkling it on your avocado toast feel like a spiritual experience. Who wouldn't be intrigued?

But here's where it gets interesting: this isn't just another baseless wellness fad. There's actually science backing up why your body responds differently to pink salt than to the processed white stuff!

Studies on electrolytes and metabolism have started catching up with what traditional healers knew for centuries. Research has found that the minerals in Himalayan pink salt help stimulate circulation and support detoxification in the body, potentially reducing bloating and water retention. Yes, that means that the post-meal puffiness you hate might actually be related to the type of salt you're using!

The fitness industry jumped on board when they realized that Himalayan pink salt can help alleviate muscle cramps by providing natural electrolytes that restore balance in the body. Suddenly, expensive sports drinks seemed unnecessary when a pinch of pink in your water could deliver minerals without the artificial junk.

Even the medical community has started paying attention. Scientific studies show that people with asthma and various respiratory conditions breathe easier after halotherapy (salt therapy), which uses microscopic salt particles to support the immune and respiratory systems.

Of course, not everyone in the scientific community is convinced. Some researchers point out that despite all the hype, there's "no evidence that pink Himalayan sea salt is healthier than regular table salt." The skeptics argue that the mineral content is too small to make a significant difference. But here's what they're missing: it's not just about the minerals. It's about choosing something less processed, more natural, and connected to ancient traditions rather than factory-produced alternatives, **and** the method of delivery.

Why It Works

Okay, so we've covered the history and origins of pink salt, but you're probably wondering if this stuff works or if it's just another wellness trend. I get it! We've all been burned by false promises before.

When regular table salt hits your system, it's just sodium chloride with some anti-caking chemicals thrown in. It's about as natural as "cheese products" that don't require refrigeration (yikes!). Your body has to work overtime just to process it, often pulling minerals from your bones and tissues just to metabolize this stripped-down salt.

But pink salt is the complete opposite. The unique combination of minerals in Himalayan salt helps "regulate the amount of water inside and outside cells, ensuring fluid balance in the body." Think about what this means for a second. Instead of bloating you up (like regular salt does), pink salt helps your cells maintain optimal hydration while flushing out what doesn't belong!

This is why people report feeling less bloated when they switch to pink salt. Unlike regular table salt, Himalayan pink salt "doesn't bind water to our tissues" due to its lower sodium content, which causes "lower water retention." Translation: The number on your scale might drop within days simply from losing excess water weight your cells have been desperately clinging to!

But the real magic happens at the metabolic level. Those 84-plus trace minerals in pink salt are the exact building blocks your body needs to fire up its fat-burning engines! The minerals in pink salt enhance cellular function, allowing the body to better absorb nutrients and flush out toxins. This can aid in weight loss by improving digestion and reducing inflammation.

Let's talk cravings for a second, you know, that 3 PM desperate hunt for anything sweet or salty that leaves you diving into office donuts? That's not a willpower issue, it's a mineral deficiency. When your body lacks essential minerals, it sends out desperate hunger signals, hoping you'll consume something that contains what it needs. Unfortunately, most processed foods just make the problem worse.

Pink salt directly tackles this problem. It can help control cravings due to its satiating property, which makes us feel full for a longer time, while also reducing insulin resistance in our bodies. Many women report that their sugar cravings virtually vanish within days of starting their pink salt ritual!

Then there's inflammation. The hidden weight loss saboteur that nobody talks about! When your body is inflamed from processed foods, stress, and environmental toxins, your cells become resistant to insulin and leptin, the hormones that regulate fat storage and hunger. The result? You store more fat and feel hungry all the time.

Pink salt is nature's anti-inflammatory superhero. By gently drawing water into the intestines, flushing out waste, reducing inflammation, and helping restore digestive flow, pink salt creates internal conditions where your body becomes more responsive to fat-burning cues. This is why people with stubborn belly fat often see the most dramatic results.

The minerals in pink salt also support your thyroid, the master control center for your metabolism. By using pink salt, you can replenish your electrolytes and hydration and improve your energy and mood, while stimulating the production of digestive enzymes and gastric juices. Without proper mineral support, your thyroid slows to a crawl, making weight loss nearly impossible no matter how little you eat or how much you exercise.

Perhaps the most fascinating aspect is how pink salt improves sleep quality. Poor sleep can increase your stress hormone cortisol, which affects your metabolism and causes you to gain weight. Many pink salt users report falling asleep faster and waking up feeling more rested, likely due to the magnesium content that helps relax muscles and calm the nervous system.

When you add it all up, better hydration, reduced cravings, decreased inflammation, improved digestion, balanced hormones, and better sleep, it's no wonder people are experiencing such dramatic results with something as simple as pink salt. And the best part? You don't need expensive equipment, complicated meal plans, or hours at the gym. Just a simple pink salt ritual that takes seconds a day, but could change your body forever. Are you ready to try it?

Chapter 2:
Facts and Myths About Pink Salt

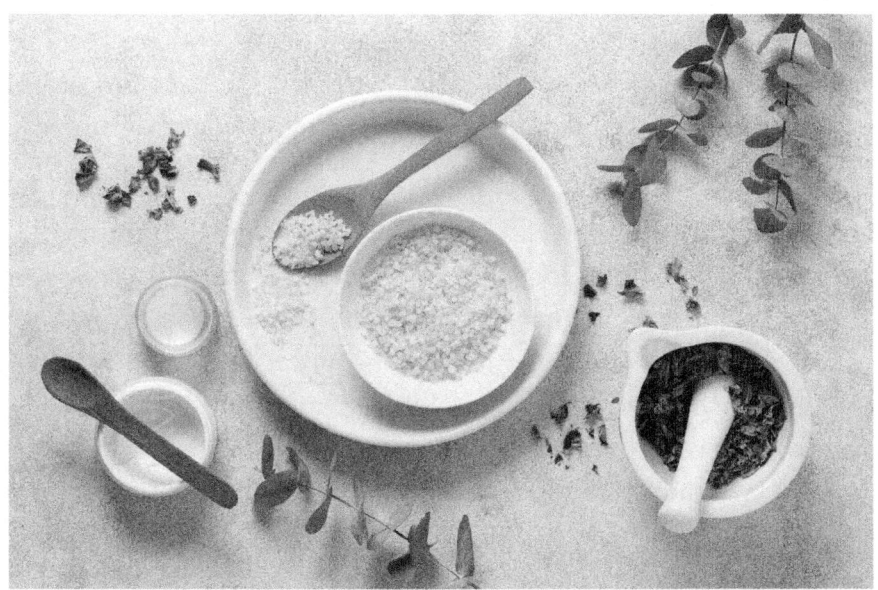

LET'S FACE IT, when something gets as popular as pink salt has, the BS factor starts rising fast! Suddenly, everyone from your yoga instructor to your mother-in-law has an opinion about this rosy crystal, and separating fact from fiction becomes nearly impossible.

I've spent years researching the truth behind pink salt, and what I've discovered might shock you. The wellness world is full of exaggerated claims about this trendy mineral, some that make me laugh out loud, and others that make me want to scream at how misleading they are.

I'm not here to crush your pink salt dreams; in fact, I'm here to let you know the truth about what it can and cannot do for you and your body. By the end of this chapter, you'll be armed with facts, not fiction, allowing you to make smart choices about how to incorporate pink salt into your wellness routine.

The truth is always more fascinating than the hype, and the real story behind pink salt is no exception.

Common Myths

Let's talk about the elephant in the salt shaker before we get to the good stuff and your pink salt trick. In my years researching this topic, I've watched wellness influencers make increasingly outlandish statements about what this pink salt can do. Some of these myths are harmless, but others might have you wasting money or, worse, making health decisions based on fiction instead of facts.

Before we dive into the real benefits of pink salt in your weight loss journey, we need to clear away the nonsense.

Myth #1: Pink Himalayan salt has less sodium than regular table salt
This is perhaps the most common misconception circulating about pink salt. The truth? Himalayan pink salt contains about 98% sodium chloride, just like regular salt. The chemical composition is virtually identical. The difference in crystal size, however, means you are receiving less sodium per serving. More importantly, you are not flooding your body with anti-caking agents or putting ultra-refined products into your body. Instead, you're receiving a good dose of minerals your body needs without the gunk.

Myth #2: Himalayan salt lamps purify the air and provide health benefits
Those pretty glowing chunks of salt have been marketed as air purifiers that release negative ions, supposedly improving everything from allergies to mood. However, scientific studies have found no scientific basis for such claimed health benefits. While they make beautiful decorative pieces that create a warm ambiance, decorative salt lamps don't measurably improve air quality or provide health benefits. If you want to reap the benefits of pink salt for better lung function, you need to use it in the way it's intended (see our chapter on holistic protocols and recipes).

Myth #3: Pink salt "detoxifies" the body
The detoxification claim appears everywhere in pink salt marketing. But here's the reality: your body already has sophisticated detoxification systems, primarily your liver and kidneys, that don't need help from salt. Scientific research confirms there is no proof to support the claim that anything detoxifies the body. What you need to do is support your body's natural detoxing process so that your body can do what it knows how to do best: eliminate itself of toxins.

Myth #4: Pink salt comes from pristine, pollution-free Himalayan mountains
The romantic image of pink salt being harvested from pristine, remote Himalayan peaks is largely marketing fiction. In reality, most pink Himalayan salt is mined from the Khewra Salt Mine in Pakistan's Punjab region. While the salt deposits were formed millions of years ago from ancient seabeds, the mining operation is industrial and modern. The salt is perfectly safe and natural, but it's not hand-harvested by monks from untouched mountain peaks as some packaging imagery might suggest.

The Science-Backed Facts

What's remarkable is that despite these myths being debunked, pink salt still offers genuine benefits when used properly, just not the magical ones often claimed in glossy advertisements.

Fact #1: Improvement in respiratory conditions
While not a miracle cure, halotherapy (salt therapy) using Himalayan salt does show promise for certain respiratory conditions. According to a 2021 study published in Alternative Therapies in

Health and Medicine, salt therapy can help relieve symptoms and improve overall function for sinusitis, bronchiectasis, chronic bronchitis, mild and moderate asthma, and even chronic obstructive pulmonary disease (COPD). The salt particles appear to have anti-inflammatory and antibacterial properties when inhaled in controlled environments.

Fact #2: Correction of electrolyte imbalances

Pink Himalayan salt contains several key electrolytes that are crucial for proper bodily function. Essential electrolytes found in pink Himalayan salt include sodium, potassium, calcium, and magnesium, which are crucial for maintaining proper fluid balance and nerve and muscle function in the body. When properly used, these minerals can support hydration and cellular function.

This is particularly relevant for active people or those who sweat heavily. Himalayan pink salt is considered ideal for hydration since it contains essential electrolytes that help regulate your fluid balance and stay hydrated. The combination of multiple minerals in one natural source makes it more comprehensive than refined salt.

Fact #3: Support for cellular function

The micronutrients in pink salt play important roles in cellular activities throughout the body. These include iron, magnesium, calcium, and potassium, which play critical roles in metabolic processes, hormonal balance, and cellular function. Each of these works synergistically to support various bodily systems.

For example, sodium from pink Himalayan salt helps your nerves send signals, your muscles contract, and assists your stomach in producing the acid it needs to digest food properly. This fundamental support for cellular communication is essential for overall health.

Fact #4: Potential anti-aging effects

Some emerging research suggests that maintaining proper mineral balance, which pink salt can support, may have anti-aging benefits. The various minerals in Himalayan salt support metabolic processes, hormonal balance, and cellular function, which are particularly beneficial for overall health.

These minerals help maintain proper hydration at the cellular level, which is key for skin health and elasticity. When cells are properly hydrated and functioning optimally, they're more resilient against the effects of aging. Additionally, the electrolyte balance supported by pink salt may help reduce inflammation, which is a key factor in premature aging.

Pink salt isn't going to transform you overnight into a swimsuit model, but (and this is a big, juicy but!) the science does back up some pretty awesome benefits that those eye-rolling skeptics love to dismiss!

While the wellness influencers might go overboard with their claims, and the science nerds might undersell it, the truth sits right in the middle; pink salt delivers real benefits when you make it part of your daily health routine.

Risks and Cautions

Pink salt can't be sprinkled on everything without a second thought. While I'm over here singing the praises of Himalayan salt, I'd be doing you a major disservice if I didn't give you the full picture. Let's talk about the potential downsides you should know about:

I don't care how pretty or mineral-rich it is, pink salt is **still** salt, which means it's packed with sodium. As medical experts consistently remind us, "Too much of any kind of salt is not good for you. Salt raises your blood pressure, which over the long term can lead to cardiovascular disease and the risk of stroke." The American Heart Association still recommends keeping your total sodium intake under 2,300mg daily, which is roughly one teaspoon of any salt, pink included.

Unlike regular table salt, which is typically fortified with iodine, pink Himalayan salt contains very little of this essential nutrient. Health experts caution that those who have iodine deficiency or are at risk of deficiency may need to source iodine elsewhere if using pink salt instead of table salt. Iodine is crucial for proper thyroid function, and deficiency can lead to serious health issues, especially during pregnancy or childhood development.

Medication Interactions

If you're on certain medications, particularly those for high blood pressure, heart conditions, or kidney issues, you need to be extra careful with **all** salt consumption. Experts warn that people who already have high blood pressure or are allergic to salt should seek guidance from their GP or other medical professional before regularly using Himalayan salt. The minerals in pink salt can interact with certain medications, so always check with your doctor.

So what's the bottom line here? Pink Himalayan salt can absolutely be part of a healthy lifestyle. Use it as you would any powerful ancient medicine, mindfully. Remember, good health comes from balance, not from going overboard with any single ingredient.

Now you know exactly what's what when it comes to pink salt: the good, the bad, and the pretty! No BS, no overblown miracle claims, just the real deal. So what are you waiting for? It's time to put this ancient mineral to work for your body!

Tomorrow morning, instead of reaching for that processed white stuff (or worse, skipping salt altogether), start your day with the Pink Salt Trick. Your cells will thank you, your taste buds will do a happy dance, and your jeans will begin fitting a little better by the end of the week.

Chapter 3:
Core Recipes Using Pink Salt

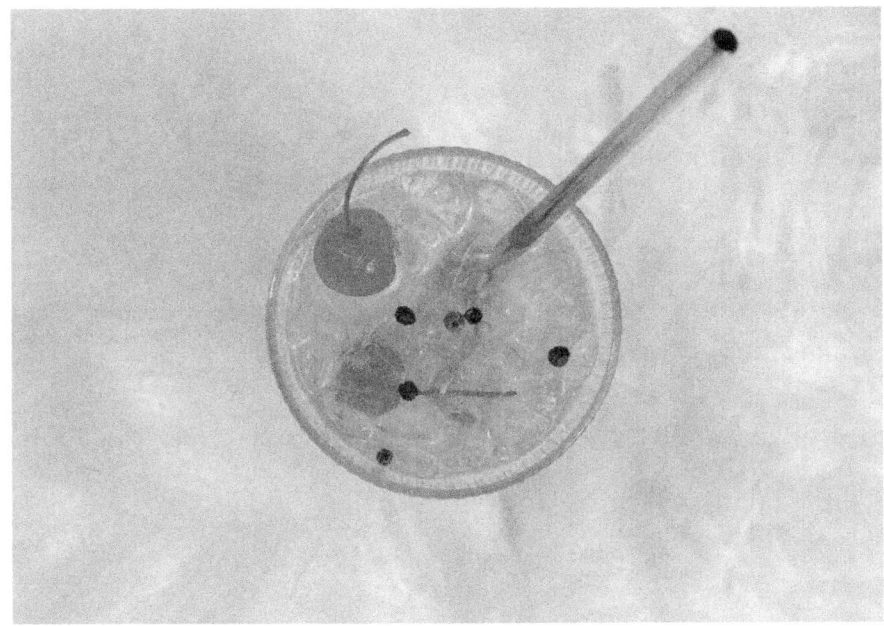

IT'S TIME TO stop talking theory and start doing something that will change your body. The Pink Salt Trick is ridiculously simple, yet the effects can be absolutely game-changing, especially if you've been battling stubborn weight, brain fog, or afternoon energy crashes that have you reaching for sugary snacks.

In this chapter, I'm going to introduce you to 30 delicious, easy-to-make recipes that turn this ancient health secret into something you'll look forward to every single day. No choking down weird-tasting concoctions or spending half your morning preparing complicated elixirs. These recipes take minutes to make but deliver benefits that last all day long.

The Classic Pink Salt Trick

Ingredients:
- 1 cup warm water
- 1/4 teaspoon Himalayan pink salt
- 1/2 fresh lemon

Instructions:
1. Warm the water to approximately 98-100°F (body temperature).

2. Add the Himalayan pink salt to the warm water and stir until completely dissolved.
3. Squeeze the fresh lemon half into the saltwater mixture.
4. If desired, stir in honey for additional flavor and potential health benefits.
5. Drink the solution immediately on an empty stomach, preferably in the morning.

Storage: Store in the refrigerator.

The Classic Pink Salt Trick Revisited

Ingredients:
- 1 cup warm water
- 1/4 teaspoon Himalayan pink salt
- 1 tablespoon raw, unfiltered apple cider vinegar

Instructions:
1. Heat water to approximately 98-100°F (body temperature).
2. Add Himalayan pink salt to the warm water and stir until completely dissolved.
3. Pour in the apple cider vinegar and mix thoroughly.
4. If using, add honey and stir until well combined.
5. Consume the drink immediately, preferably on an empty stomach in the morning.

Storage: Consume immediately after preparation.

Recipe Variations

Metabolism Mixer

Ingredients:
- 1 cup filtered water
- ¼ teaspoon Himalayan pink salt
- 1 tablespoon brewed green tea
- ½ teaspoon raw honey
- 2 crushed peppermint leaves
- Ice cubes

Instructions:
1. Brew green tea using hot water and steep for 3-4 minutes.
2. Remove the tea bag and allow the tea to cool to room temperature, approximately 15-20 minutes.
3. Sprinkle Himalayan pink salt over the cooled tea and stir until completely dissolved.
4. Finely chop fresh peppermint leaves.
5. Add chopped peppermint leaves to tea.
6. Drizzle honey and mix thoroughly until well incorporated.
7. Add 3-4 ice cubes to chill the drink.

8. Stir gently to ensure even temperature and flavor distribution.
9. Serve immediately.

Storage: Store in the fridge for up to 48 hours in a sealed glass jar.

Aloe Vera Elixir

Ingredients:
- ½ cup pure aloe vera juice (unsweetened)
- ½ cup filtered water
- ¼ teaspoon Himalayan pink salt
- 1 tablespoon fresh lime juice
- 3 fresh mint leaves
- ½ teaspoon raw honey

Instructions:
1. Pour aloe vera juice and water into a clean glass.
2. Gently tear fresh mint leaves by hand to release essential oils.
3. Add torn mint leaves to the liquid mixture.
4. Cut the lime in half and squeeze fresh juice directly into the glass.
5. Sprinkle Himalayan pink salt evenly across the surface.
6. Drizzle honey into the mixture.
7. Stir thoroughly for 20-30 seconds to ensure all ingredients are well combined.
8. Add 2-3 ice cubes to chill the drink.
9. Serve immediately.

Storage: Store in the fridge for up to **48 hours**.

Hydration Blend

Ingredients:
- 1 cup coconut water
- ¼ teaspoon Himalayan pink salt
- 1 tablespoon chia seeds
- 3 fresh basil leaves
- ½ teaspoon liquid chlorophyll
- Ice cubes

Instructions:
1. Pour coconut water into a clean glass.
2. Sprinkle Himalayan pink salt evenly over the surface.
3. Stir thoroughly until salt is completely dissolved.
4. Add chia seeds to coconut water.
5. Allow seeds to soak for 10-15 minutes, stirring occasionally to prevent clumping.

Wind Electrolyte Fusion

Ingredients:
- 3/4 cup coconut water
- 1/4 cup cucumber juice
- 1/4 teaspoon Himalayan pink salt
- 1 tablespoon lime juice
- 2 drops of liquid stevia
- Fresh rosemary sprig

Instructions:
1. Wash cucumber thoroughly and trim ends.
2. Cut cucumber into chunks suitable for blending.
3. Using a blender, process the cucumber until smooth.
4. Strain cucumber juice through a fine-mesh sieve.
5. Pour coconut water into a clean glass.
6. Add fresh cucumber juice to coconut water.
7. Sprinkle Himalayan pink salt evenly across the surface.
8. Stir thoroughly for 15-20 seconds to dissolve salt.
9. Cut the lime in half and squeeze fresh juice directly into the mixture.
10. Add liquid stevia, starting with a small amount.
11. Stir for 20-30 seconds to ensure even distribution.
12. Gently wash a fresh rosemary sprig.
13. Garnish the glass with a rosemary sprig.
14. Serve immediately.

Storage: Store for up to **24 hours** in a sealed glass jar to preserve nutrients.

Crystalline Cleanse

Ingredients:
- 1 cup chamomile tea (cooled)
- ¼ teaspoon Himalayan pink salt
- 1 tablespoon lemon juice
- ½ teaspoon raw agave nectar
- Thin lemon slice
- Tiny pinch of grated fresh ginger

Instructions:
1. Boil water and steep a chamomile tea bag for 3-4 minutes.
2. Remove the tea bag and allow the tea to cool to room temperature, approximately 10-15 minutes.
3. Pour cooled tea into a clean glass.

4. Sprinkle Himalayan pink salt evenly across the surface.
5. Stir thoroughly for 15-20 seconds to completely dissolve the salt.
6. Cut the lemon in half and squeeze fresh juice directly into the tea.
7. Measure agave nectar and drizzle into the mixture.
8. Grate fresh ginger using a microplane.
9. Add grated ginger to the tea.
10. Stir for 20-30 seconds to ensure even distribution of ingredients.
11. Cut a thin lemon slice for garnish.
12. Garnish the glass with a lemon slice.
13. Serve at room temperature.

Storage: Store in the fridge for **up to 24 hours**.

Surge Hydro-Blend

Ingredients:
- 3/4 cup kombucha
- 1/4 cup pomegranate juice
- 1/4 teaspoon Himalayan pink salt
- 1 tablespoon chia seeds
- 2 drops of liquid monk fruit sweetener
- Fresh thyme sprig

Instructions:
1. Pour kombucha into a clean glass.
2. Add pomegranate juice to kombucha.
3. Sprinkle Himalayan pink salt evenly across the surface.
4. Stir thoroughly for 15-20 seconds to completely dissolve the salt.
5. Measure chia seeds carefully.
6. Sprinkle chia seeds over the mixture, stirring immediately to prevent clumping.
7. Let the mixture sit for 10-15 minutes to allow chia seeds to begin absorbing liquid.
8. Add monk fruit sweetener, starting with a small amount.
9. Stir for 20-30 seconds to ensure even distribution.
10. Gently wash a fresh thyme sprig.
11. Pluck a few fresh thyme leaves.
12. Garnish the glass with thyme leaves.
13. Add 2-3 ice cubes to chill.
14. Stir gently before serving.

Storage: Can be stored for **24 hours** max (due to kombucha fizz and chia).

Recovery Drink

Ingredients:
- 1 cup cold brew green tea
- ¼ teaspoon Himalayan pink salt
- ½ teaspoon turmeric powder
- 1 pinch ground black pepper
- ½ teaspoon raw honey
- Thin orange slice

Instructions:
1. Brew green tea and allow it to cool to room temperature.
2. Pour cooled green tea into a clean glass.
3. Sift ground turmeric powder into tea to prevent clumping.
4. Add ground black pepper.
5. Whisk thoroughly for 20-30 seconds to ensure complete incorporation.
6. Sprinkle Himalayan pink salt evenly across the surface.
7. Stir for 15-20 seconds to dissolve salt completely.
8. Drizzle honey into the mixture.
9. Stir for 20-30 seconds to ensure even distribution.
10. Cut a thin orange slice for garnish.
11. Garnish the glass with an orange slice.
12. Serve at room temperature.

Storage: Store up to **24 hours** in a glass jar.

Rejuvenation Liquid

Ingredients:
- 3/4 cup beetroot juice
- 1/4 cup coconut water
- 1/4 teaspoon Himalayan pink salt
- 1 tablespoon ginger juice
- 2 drops of liquid stevia
- Fresh mint leaves

Instructions:
1. Juice fresh beetroot using a juicer or blender.
2. Strain beetroot juice through a fine-mesh sieve.
3. Pour coconut water into a clean glass.
4. Add fresh beetroot juice to coconut water.
5. Sprinkle Himalayan pink salt evenly across the surface.
6. Stir thoroughly for 15-20 seconds to completely dissolve the salt.

7. Grate fresh ginger using a microplane.
8. Press grated ginger through a fine-mesh sieve to extract juice.
9. Add fresh ginger juice to the mixture.
10. Add liquid stevia, starting with a small amount.
11. Stir for 20-30 seconds to ensure even distribution.
12. Gently tear fresh mint leaves by hand to release essential oils.
13. Add torn mint leaves to the mixture.
14. Add 2-3 ice cubes to chill.
15. Stir gently before serving.

Storage: Store up to **48 hours** in the fridge. Shake well before use.

Energy Infusion

Ingredients:
- 1 cup hibiscus tea (cooled)
- ¼ teaspoon Himalayan pink salt
- 1 tablespoon elderberry syrup
- ½ teaspoon raw maple syrup
- Edible flower petals (optional garnish)

Instructions:
1. Brew hibiscus tea using hot water and steep for 3-4 minutes.
2. Remove the tea bag and allow the tea to cool to room temperature, approximately 10-15 minutes.
3. Pour cooled tea into a clean glass.
4. Sprinkle Himalayan pink salt evenly across the surface.
5. Stir thoroughly for 15-20 seconds to completely dissolve the salt.
6. Add elderberry syrup to tea.
7. Drizzle maple syrup into the mixture.
8. Stir for 20-30 seconds to ensure even distribution.
9. Gently wash fresh mint leaves.
10. Tear mint leaves by hand to release essential oils.
11. Garnish the glass with torn mint leaves.
12. Add 1-2 ice cubes if desired.
13. Serve at room temperature.

Storage: Store in the fridge for **up to 48 hours**.

Rhythm Replenisher

Ingredients:
- 3/4 cup kefir water
- 1/4 cup passion fruit juice

- 1/4 teaspoon Himalayan pink salt
- 1 tablespoon maca powder
- 2 drops vanilla stevia
- Fresh passionfruit seeds

Instructions:
1. Pour kefir water into a clean glass.
2. Add fresh passion fruit juice to kefir water.
3. Sprinkle Himalayan pink salt evenly across the surface.
4. Stir thoroughly for 15-20 seconds to completely dissolve the salt.
5. Sift maca powder into the mixture to prevent clumping.
6. Whisk for 30-45 seconds to ensure complete incorporation.
7. Add vanilla stevia, starting with a small amount.
8. Stir for 20-30 seconds to ensure even distribution.
9. Cut fresh passion fruit in half.
10. Scoop out passionfruit seeds directly into the mixture.
11. Stir gently to distribute seeds.
12. Add 2-3 ice cubes to chill.
13. Serve immediately.

Storage: Store up to **24 hours** in the fridge (probiotics degrade with time).

Mineral Mist

Ingredients:
- 1 cup watermelon juice
- ¼ teaspoon Himalayan pink salt
- 1 teaspoon activated charcoal powder
- ½ teaspoon raw honey
- Thin cucumber ribbon

Instructions:
1. Pour fresh watermelon juice into a clean glass.
2. Sprinkle Himalayan pink salt evenly across the surface.
3. Stir thoroughly for 15-20 seconds to completely dissolve the salt.
4. Sift activated charcoal powder into the mixture to prevent clumping.
5. Whisk for 30-45 seconds to ensure complete incorporation.
6. Drizzle honey into the mixture.
7. Stir for 20-30 seconds to ensure even distribution.
8. Wash the cucumber thoroughly.
9. Cut cucumber into thin ribbons using a vegetable peeler.
10. Garnish the glass with cucumber ribbon.
11. Add 2-3 ice cubes to chill.

12. Serve immediately.

Storage: Best consumed within **12 hours** (charcoal can settle unevenly).

Vitality Elixir

Ingredients:
- 3/4 cup green coconut water
- 1/4 cup dragon fruit juice
- 1/4 teaspoon Himalayan pink salt
- 1 tablespoon spirulina powder
- 2 drops of liquid monk fruit sweetener
- Fresh basil leaves

Instructions:
1. Pour green coconut water into a blender.
2. Cut dragon fruit in half and scoop flesh into a blender.
3. Blend for 30-45 seconds until smooth.
4. Pour the blended mixture into a clean glass.
5. Sprinkle Himalayan pink salt evenly across the surface.
6. Stir thoroughly for 15-20 seconds to completely dissolve the salt.
7. Sift spirulina powder into the mixture to prevent clumping.
8. Whisk for 30-45 seconds to ensure complete incorporation.
9. Add monk fruit sweetener, starting with a small amount.
10. Stir for 20-30 seconds to ensure even distribution.
11. Gently tear fresh basil leaves by hand to release essential oils.
12. Add torn basil leaves to the mixture.
13. Add 2-3 ice cubes to chill.
14. Serve immediately.

Storage: Best within **24 hours**, especially due to spirulina and fresh herbs.

Traditional Drinks

Ayurvedic Salt Lassi

Ingredients:
- 1 cup fresh yogurt
- 1/2 cup cold water
- 1/4 teaspoon Himalayan pink salt
- 1/2 teaspoon cumin powder
- Fresh mint leaves
- Pinch of black pepper

Instructions:
1. Whisk yogurt until smooth.
2. Gradually add water and continue whisking.
3. Sprinkle Himalayan pink salt and cumin powder.
4. Stir until completely integrated.
5. Garnish with fresh mint leaves and black pepper.
6. Serve chilled.

Storage: Consume within 2 hours, refrigerated.

Electrolyte Pink Salt Broth

Ingredients:
- 2 cups bone broth
- 1/2 teaspoon Himalayan pink salt
- 1 tablespoon fresh parsley
- 1 small piece of ginger
- 1 clove roasted garlic
- Pinch of turmeric

Instructions:
1. Pour bone broth into a medium saucepan.
2. Heat bone broth over a low flame, stirring occasionally to prevent scorching.
3. Remove from heat once broth is warm, not boiling.
4. Pour warm broth into a clean serving mug.
5. Sprinkle Himalayan pink salt evenly across the surface.
6. Stir thoroughly for 15-20 seconds to completely dissolve the salt.
7. Finely chop fresh parsley using a sharp knife.
8. Grate fresh ginger using a microplane.
9. Add minced parsley and grated ginger to the broth.
10. Crush the roasted garlic clove and add to the mixture.
11. Sprinkle ground turmeric over the top.
12. Stir gently to incorporate all ingredients.
13. Serve immediately while warm.

Storage: Refrigerate and consume within 3 days.

Sole Water

Ingredients:
- 1 cup filtered water
- 1 teaspoon Himalayan pink salt brine (concentrated salt solution)
- 1 slice of lemon

- Fresh thyme sprig
- Optional: 1 tablespoon fresh cucumber juice

Instructions:
1. In a clean glass jar, combine filtered water and Himalayan pink salt.
2. Stir thoroughly until salt is completely dissolved.
3. Cover the jar with a clean cloth or a loose lid.
4. Allow brine to sit at room temperature for 24 hours.
5. After 24 hours, strain the brine through a fine-mesh sieve.
6. Store concentrated salt solution in a clean, sealed glass container.
7. Pour fresh water into a drinking glass.
8. Measure exactly 1 teaspoon of salt brine.
9. Add brine to water and stir for 15-20 seconds.
10. Cut fresh lemon into thin slices.
11. Squeeze the lemon slice directly into water.
12. Gently wash a fresh thyme sprig.
13. Garnish the glass with a thyme sprig.
14. Serve immediately.

Storage: Concentrated salt brine can be stored at room temperature for up to 1 month. The prepared drink should be consumed immediately.

Masala Soda

Ingredients:
- 1 cup sparkling water
- 1/4 teaspoon Himalayan pink salt
- 1/2 teaspoon roasted cumin powder
- Fresh mint leaves
- 1/2 lime, juiced
- Pinch of chaat masala

Instructions:
1. Open a bottle of sparkling water.
2. Pour sparkling water into a clean glass.
3. Sprinkle Himalayan pink salt evenly across the surface.
4. Stir thoroughly for 15-20 seconds to dissolve salt.
5. Measure roasted cumin powder.
6. Sprinkle roasted cumin powder over the mixture.
7. Cut fresh lime in half.
8. Squeeze lime juice directly into the glass.
9. Add a pinch of chaat masala.
10. Stir for 20-30 seconds to ensure even distribution.

11. Gently wash fresh mint leaves.
12. Tear mint leaves by hand to release essential oils.
13. Garnish the glass with torn mint leaves.
14. Serve immediately.

Storage: Best consumed immediately to maintain carbonation.

Golden Milk Salt Tonic

Ingredients:
- 1 cup fresh whole milk
- 1/4 teaspoon Himalayan pink salt
- 1 tablespoon fresh turmeric root, grated
- 1/2 teaspoon ground cinnamon
- Pinch of black pepper
- Small piece of fresh ginger, grated

Instructions:
1. Pour fresh whole milk into a medium saucepan.
2. Heat milk over a low flame, stirring occasionally to prevent scorching.
3. Remove from heat just before the milk reaches a boil.
4. Sprinkle Himalayan pink salt evenly across the surface of the milk.
5. Stir thoroughly for 15-20 seconds to dissolve salt.
6. Using a microplane, grate fresh turmeric root.
7. Grate fresh ginger root.
8. Add grated turmeric and ginger to warm milk.
9. Sprinkle ground cinnamon over the surface.
10. Add a pinch of freshly ground black pepper.
11. Whisk continuously for 30-45 seconds to fully incorporate ingredients.
12. Place a fine-mesh strainer over a serving mug.
13. Pour the milk mixture through a strainer to remove ginger and turmeric fibers.
14. Serve immediately while warm.

Storage: Consume within 2 hours, best served immediately.

Mineral Bone Broth Elixir

Ingredients:
- 2 cups homemade beef bone broth
- 1/2 teaspoon Himalayan pink salt
- 1 tablespoon fresh parsley
- 1 small piece of kombu seaweed
- 1 egg yolk

- Fresh thyme sprig

Instructions:
1. Pour bone broth into a medium saucepan.
2. Heat bone broth over a low flame, stirring occasionally to prevent scorching.
3. Remove from heat just before the broth reaches a boil.
4. Sprinkle Himalayan pink salt evenly across the surface.
5. Stir thoroughly for 15-20 seconds to dissolve salt.
6. Rinse kombu seaweed under cold water.
7. Add kombu seaweed to warm broth.
8. Let seaweed steep for exactly 5 minutes.
9. Remove kombu seaweed using a slotted spoon.
10. Separate egg yolk from white, keeping the yolk intact.
11. Gently whisk raw egg yolk into broth.
12. Finely chop fresh parsley.
13. Pluck fresh thyme leaves.
14. Garnish with chopped parsley and thyme leaves.
15. Serve immediately.

Storage: Consume within 24 hours, refrigerate promptly.

Turmeric Salt Chai

Ingredients:
- 1 cup fresh whole milk
- 1/4 teaspoon Himalayan pink salt
- 1 tablespoon fresh turmeric root
- 2 cardamom pods
- 1 small cinnamon stick
- Fresh ginger slice
- 1 whole clove

Instructions:
1. Using the flat side of a knife, gently crush cardamom pods to release seeds.
2. Break the cinnamon stick into smaller pieces using your hands.
3. Pour fresh whole milk into a medium saucepan.
4. Add crushed cardamom pods and cinnamon stick pieces to the milk.
5. Heat milk over a low flame, stirring occasionally.
6. Sprinkle Himalayan pink salt evenly across the surface.
7. Simmer gently for exactly 10 minutes, avoiding boiling.
8. Remove from heat.
9. Place a fine-mesh strainer over a serving mug.
10. Pour the milk mixture through a strainer to remove spices.

12. Cut a thin cucumber slice.
13. Garnish the glass with a cucumber slice.
14. Add 2-3 ice cubes to chill.
15. Stir gently before serving.

Storage: Refrigerate and consume within 24 hours.

Tips for Success

You've got the recipes, but let's talk about how to make this Pink Salt Trick your own so you'll actually stick with it long enough to see results!

Not everyone's palate is the same, and that's totally okay! If the classic morning pink salt drink is too salty for your taste, start with just a pinch and gradually increase to the full amount as your taste buds adjust. Can't stand lemon? Swap in lime or a splash of cranberry juice instead. The key is making something you'll actually drink every morning, not something that makes you gag!

For maximum metabolic benefits, try to have your Pink Salt Trick drink first thing in the morning, ideally 30 minutes before eating anything. This gives the minerals time to wake up your digestive enzymes and get your metabolism humming before food enters the picture. But if mornings are crazy for you, don't stress, having it a bit later is still way better than skipping it altogether!

If you're watching your sugar intake or following a keto/low-carb lifestyle, you can absolutely make these recipes work for you! Skip the honey in the classic recipe and try a few drops of liquid stevia or monk fruit extract instead. They provide sweetness without the glucose spike that can interfere with fat-burning. For fruity variations, use just a small amount of berries or swap in sugar-free extracts for flavor.

Hormone-Friendly Modifications

Ladies dealing with hormone fluctuations (hello, perimenopause!) might benefit from adding adaptogenic herbs to their Pink Salt drinks. A quarter teaspoon of maca powder or ashwagandha can help balance those hormonal roller coasters without changing the taste dramatically. During PMS weeks, adding a little extra magnesium (in the form of a powdered supplement) to your drink can help reduce bloating and cramps!

While room temperature water is ideal for absorption, some people just can't handle lukewarm drinks first thing in the morning. If you need your morning ritual to be cold and refreshing, prepare your Pink Salt drink the night before and refrigerate it. For those who prefer something warm and cozy, especially in winter months, you can use warm (not boiling) water, just be sure to dissolve the salt completely before adding other ingredients.

Don't just gulp it down while racing around getting ready! Take 30 seconds to sip mindfully, imagining those minerals energizing your cells and firing up your fat-burning engines. This tiny moment of mindfulness not only enhances the physical benefits but also sets a positive tone for making healthy choices throughout the rest of your day.

The time for thinking, wondering, and questioning is over. Tomorrow morning, instead of reaching for that phone to check social media the second your eyes open, make the classic Pink Salt Trick recipe your very first act of the day!

- 1/2 teaspoon Himalayan pink salt
- 1 tablespoon olive oil
- Fresh rosemary
- Cayenne pepper (optional)

Instructions:
1. Place a large skillet over medium heat and allow it to warm for 1-2 minutes.
2. Add mixed nuts (almonds, cashews, walnuts) to the dry skillet and toast for 2-3 minutes, stirring constantly to prevent burning.
3. Drizzle olive oil evenly over the toasted nuts, ensuring all are lightly coated.
4. Sprinkle Himalayan pink salt evenly across the nuts.
5. Finely chop fresh rosemary and scatter over the nuts.
6. Quickly toss the nuts to distribute oil, salt, and rosemary, then immediately remove the skillet from the heat to prevent over-toasting.

Storage: Store in an airtight container for up to 5 days.

No-Cook Seed Sprinkle Crunch

Ingredients:
- 1/2 cup raw pumpkin seeds
- 1/2 cup sunflower seeds
- 1/4 cup chia seeds
- 1/4 teaspoon Himalayan pink salt
- 2 tablespoons nutritional yeast
- 1 tablespoon olive oil

Instructions:
1. In a large mixing bowl, combine pumpkin seeds, sunflower seeds, and chia seeds, stirring to evenly distribute the different seed types.
2. Drizzle olive oil evenly over the seeds, using just enough to lightly coat them without creating pools of oil.
3. Sprinkle Himalayan pink salt evenly across the seed mixture.
4. Add nutritional yeast over the seeds, ensuring even distribution.
5. Using a spatula or large spoon, toss the seeds thoroughly to ensure every seed is coated with oil, salt, and nutritional yeast.
6. Transfer to a serving bowl and enjoy immediately as a crunchy topping for salads, yogurt, or as a standalone snack.

Storage: Store in an airtight container for up to 1 week.

Egg Salt Boats

Ingredients:
- 3 hard-boiled eggs
- 1/4 teaspoon Himalayan pink salt
- 2 tablespoons Greek yogurt
- Fresh chives
- Smoked paprika
- Cracked black pepper

Instructions:
1. Carefully slice hard-boiled eggs in half lengthwise using a sharp knife, wiping the blade clean between cuts to ensure neat halves.
2. Gently remove egg yolks and place them in a small mixing bowl. Mash the yolks thoroughly with a fork.
3. Add Greek yogurt to the mashed yolks and mix until smooth and well combined.
4. Sprinkle Himalayan pink salt evenly into the yolk-yogurt mixture, stirring to incorporate.
5. Using a small spoon, carefully fill each egg white half with the prepared yogurt mixture, mounding slightly.
6. Finely chop fresh chives and sprinkle over the filled eggs.
7. Dust the top of each egg with smoked paprika for added flavor and color.
8. Arrange on a serving plate and serve immediately.

Storage: Refrigerate and consume within 24 hours.

Quickest Cheese Crisp Medley

Ingredients:
- 1 cup mixed cheese (cheddar, parmesan)
- 1/4 teaspoon Himalayan pink salt
- Fresh thyme leaves
- Cracked black pepper
- Parchment paper

Instructions:
1. Preheat the oven to 400°F and line a rimmed baking sheet with parchment paper.
2. Using a grater or cheese slicer, create small, thin circles of cheese, spacing them about 1 inch apart on the prepared baking sheet.
3. Sprinkle a light, even layer of Himalayan pink salt over each cheese circle.
4. Place the baking sheet in the preheated oven and bake for 3-5 minutes, watching carefully to prevent burning.
5. Remove the baking sheet from the oven when the cheese circles' edges are golden brown and crisp.

6. Let the cheese crisps cool for 1-2 minutes, then carefully transfer to a serving plate.
7. Garnish with fresh thyme leaves and a light sprinkle of freshly cracked black pepper.

Storage: Consume immediately for maximum crispness.

Super Speed Veggie Salt Dip

Ingredients:
- 1/2 cup Greek yogurt
- 1/4 teaspoon Himalayan pink salt
- 2 tablespoons fresh dill
- 1 clove minced garlic
- 1 tablespoon lemon juice
- Cracked black pepper

Instructions:
1. In a medium mixing bowl, place Greek yogurt, allowing it to come to slightly cool room temperature for easier mixing.
2. Sprinkle Himalayan pink salt evenly over the surface of the yogurt.
3. Finely mince fresh dill and garlic using a sharp knife, creating small, uniform pieces.
4. Cut a fresh lemon in half and squeeze juice directly into the yogurt, being careful to catch any seeds.
5. Using a whisk or spatula, mix all ingredients thoroughly, ensuring the salt, dill, garlic, and lemon juice are completely incorporated into the Greek yogurt.
6. Transfer the dip to a serving bowl and arrange an assortment of raw vegetable sticks around the edge for dipping.

Storage: Refrigerate and consume within 3 days.

Instant Protein Power Bites

Ingredients:
- 1 cup rolled oats
- 1/2 cup almond butter
- 1/4 cup chia seeds
- 1/4 teaspoon Himalayan pink salt
- 2 tablespoons honey
- 1/4 cup dark chocolate chips

Instructions:
1. In a large mixing bowl, combine rolled oats, almond butter, chia seeds, and protein powder, stirring until the ingredients are well mixed.
2. Add honey to the mixture and mix thoroughly until the ingredients hold together when pressed.

3. Using clean hands, roll the mixture into uniform, small bite-sized balls, approximately 1-inch in diameter.
4. Lightly sprinkle Himalayan pink salt over the surface of each energy bite.
5. Gently press 2-3 dark chocolate chips into the top of each bite, ensuring they adhere to the surface.
6. Place the energy bites on a parchment-lined tray and refrigerate for 10 minutes to help them set.
7. Serve chilled directly from the refrigerator.

Storage: Refrigerate up to 1 week in a sealed container.

Zero-Prep Roasted Seed Scatter

Ingredients:
- 1/2 cup pumpkin seeds
- 1/2 cup sunflower seeds
- 1/4 teaspoon Himalayan pink salt
- 1 tablespoon olive oil
- Fresh rosemary
- Smoked paprika

Instructions:
1. In a large, dry skillet, combine pumpkin seeds and sunflower seeds, spreading them in an even layer.
2. Drizzle olive oil evenly over the seeds, using just enough to lightly coat them.
3. Sprinkle Himalayan pink salt evenly across the seeds.
4. Toast the seeds over medium heat, stirring constantly to prevent burning, for approximately 3-4 minutes or until seeds are golden and fragrant.
5. Remove skillet from heat and immediately sprinkle fresh chopped rosemary and smoked paprika over the toasted seeds.
6. Toss the seeds quickly to distribute herbs and spices, then transfer to a serving dish.

Storage: Store in an airtight container for 5 days.

Frozen Yogurt Salt Clusters

Ingredients:
- 2 cups Greek yogurt
- 1/4 teaspoon Himalayan pink salt
- 2 tablespoons honey
- 1/4 cup mixed berries
- 2 tablespoons chopped almonds
- Parchment paper

Instructions:
1. Line a rimmed baking sheet with parchment paper, ensuring the paper is flat and smooth.
2. In a medium mixing bowl, combine Greek yogurt and honey, stirring until well blended and smooth.
3. Sprinkle Himalayan pink salt evenly over the yogurt mixture, stirring gently to incorporate.
4. Using a tablespoon, drop small dollops of the yogurt mixture onto the prepared baking sheet, spacing them about 1 inch apart.
5. Sprinkle a mix of fresh berries and chopped almonds over each yogurt cluster.
6. Place the baking sheet in the freezer for 30-45 minutes, or until the yogurt clusters are completely firm to the touch.

Storage: Keep frozen, consume within 1 week.

Anti-Inflammatory On-the-Go Foods

Turmeric Protein Power Balls

Ingredients:
- 1 cup almond flour
- 1/2 cup plant-based protein powder
- 2 tablespoons ground turmeric
- 1/4 teaspoon Himalayan pink salt
- 1/4 cup almond butter
- 3 tablespoons raw honey
- 2 tablespoons ground flaxseed

Instructions:
1. In a large mixing bowl, combine almond flour, plant-based protein powder, ground turmeric, and ground flaxseed, whisking to ensure even distribution.
2. Create a well in the center of the dry ingredients and add almond butter and honey.
3. Using clean hands, knead the ingredients together until a uniform, slightly sticky dough forms.
4. Roll the mixture between your palms to create small, uniform bite-sized balls, approximately 1-inch in diameter.
5. Place the balls on a parchment-lined tray and refrigerate for 30 minutes to allow them to firm up.
6. Transfer the protein balls to an airtight container, separating layers with parchment paper to prevent sticking.

Storage: Refrigerate up to 1 week.

Ginger Overnight Oats

Ingredients:
- 1/2 cup rolled oats
- 1/2 cup almond milk
- 1 tablespoon fresh grated ginger
- 1/4 teaspoon Himalayan pink salt
- 2 tablespoons chia seeds
- 1 tablespoon maple syrup
- Fresh berries for topping

Instructions:
1. In a medium-sized mason jar or container, combine rolled oats and almond milk, stirring to ensure oats are fully submerged.
2. Grate fresh ginger using a microplane or fine grater directly into the oat mixture, distributing evenly.
3. Sprinkle Himalayan pink salt over the surface and stir to incorporate.
4. Add chia seeds and maple syrup, mixing thoroughly to prevent clumping.
5. Securely cover the container and place it in the refrigerator for at least 8 hours or overnight.
6. Before serving, give the overnight oats a good stir. Top with a variety of fresh berries such as blueberries, raspberries, or sliced strawberries.

Storage: Refrigerate up to 3 days.

Omega-3 Chia Cups

Ingredients:
- 1/4 cup chia seeds
- 1 cup coconut milk
- 2 tablespoons ground flaxseed
- 1/4 teaspoon Himalayan pink salt
- 1 tablespoon honey
- Fresh blueberries
- Chopped walnuts

Instructions:
1. In a medium mixing bowl, combine chia seeds and coconut milk, stirring thoroughly to prevent clumping.
2. Sprinkle ground flaxseed over the chia and coconut milk mixture, whisking to ensure even distribution.
3. Add Himalayan pink salt, stirring gently to incorporate.
4. Drizzle honey over the mixture and stir until well combined.

5. Cover the bowl and let it sit at room temperature for 15 minutes, stirring occasionally. The mixture will thicken and develop a pudding-like consistency.
6. Once thickened, transfer the mixture to serving cups or glasses.
7. Top each serving with fresh blueberries and chopped walnuts, distributing evenly.

Storage: Refrigerate up to 3 days.

Blueberry Bites

Ingredients:
- 1 cup rolled oats
- 1/2 cup dried blueberries
- 1/4 cup almond butter
- 2 tablespoons hemp seeds
- 1/4 teaspoon Himalayan pink salt
- 3 tablespoons raw honey
- 1/4 cup dark chocolate chips

Instructions:
1. In a large mixing bowl, combine rolled oats and dried blueberries, stirring to evenly distribute the blueberries.
2. Add almond butter to the oat mixture and mix thoroughly until the almond butter is well incorporated.
3. Sprinkle hemp seeds over the mixture and fold in gently.
4. Sprinkle Himalayan pink salt evenly across the mixture.
5. Drizzle honey over the ingredients and mix until the mixture holds together when pressed.
6. Using clean hands, roll the mixture into small, uniform bite-sized balls, about 1 inch in diameter.
7. Gently press 2-3 dark chocolate chips onto the top of each energy bite.

Storage: Refrigerate up to 1 week.

Salmon Omega Prep Rolls

Ingredients:
- 2 sheets of nori seaweed
- 4 oz smoked salmon
- 1/4 cup cream cheese
- 1/4 teaspoon Himalayan pink salt
- Fresh dill
- Cucumber strips
- Lemon zest

Instructions:
1. Place two nori seaweed sheets on a clean cutting board, shiny side down.
2. Using a butter knife or small spatula, spread an even layer of cream cheese across each sheet, leaving a 1/2-inch border at the top edge.
3. Arrange smoked salmon strips in a single layer over the cream cheese, covering about 2/3 of the sheet.
4. Sprinkle Himalayan pink salt evenly over the salmon.
5. Thinly slice cucumber into matchstick-sized strips and chop fresh dill.
6. Distribute cucumber strips and chopped dill evenly over the salmon.
7. Starting from the bottom edge, carefully roll the nori sheet tightly, using the bare top edge to seal the roll.
8. Using a sharp knife, slice the roll into 6-8 bite-sized pieces.

Storage: Refrigerate up to 3 days.

Green Tea Protein Cups

Ingredients:
- 1 scoop vanilla protein powder
- 1 tablespoon matcha powder
- 1/2 cup Greek yogurt
- 1/4 teaspoon Himalayan pink salt
- 2 tablespoons honey
- Chopped pistachios
- Fresh mint leaves

Instructions:
1. In a medium mixing bowl, combine protein powder and matcha powder, whisking until no lumps remain.
2. Add Greek yogurt to the powder mixture and stir thoroughly until completely smooth and well blended.
3. Sprinkle Himalayan pink salt over the mixture and gently fold in.
4. Drizzle honey into the mixture and stir until evenly incorporated.
5. Carefully spoon or pour the mixture into silicone cups, filling each cup about 3/4 full.
6. Chop pistachios and tear fresh mint leaves, then sprinkle over the top of each cup.

Storage: Refrigerate up to 3 days.

Superfood Smoothie Packs

Ingredients:
- 2 1/2 cups frozen spinach
- 1 1/4 cups frozen pineapple

- 10 tablespoons of goji berries
- 5 tablespoons turmeric powder
- 1 1/4 teaspoons Himalayan pink salt
- 5 scoops of collagen powder
- 5 zip-lock freezer bags

Instructions:
1. Prepare 5 individual zip-lock freezer bags.
2. In each bag, measure 1/2 cup frozen spinach, 1/4 cup frozen pineapple, 2 tablespoons goji berries, 1 tablespoon turmeric powder, 1/4 teaspoon Himalayan pink salt, and 1 scoop collagen powder.
3. Seal bags completely, removing excess air.
4. Label bags with contents and date.
5. Freeze immediately.

Blending Instructions:
1. Empty one smoothie pack into a blender.
2. Add 1 cup coconut water.
3. Blend for 45-60 seconds until smooth.
4. Serve immediately.

Storage: Freezer packs last up to 1 month. Each pack makes one 12-oz smoothie.

Walnut Breakfast Clusters

Ingredients:
- 1 cup raw walnuts
- 1/2 cup rolled oats
- 2 tablespoons ground flaxseed
- 1/4 teaspoon Himalayan pink salt
- 3 tablespoons raw honey
- 1 teaspoon cinnamon
- Dried tart cherries

Instructions:
1. Preheat oven to 350°F (175°C).
2. Spread walnuts in a single layer on a baking sheet.
3. Toast walnuts for 8-10 minutes, stirring once halfway through.
4. Remove from oven and let cool for 5 minutes.
5. Chop toasted walnuts into smaller pieces.
6. In a large mixing bowl, combine chopped walnuts, rolled oats, and ground flaxseed.
7. Sprinkle Himalayan pink salt over the mixture.
8. Warm honey slightly to make it more liquid.

9. Add cinnamon to the honey and mix.
10. Pour the honey mixture over the dry ingredients.
11. Stir until all ingredients are well-coated.
12. Press mixture into a lined 8x8-inch baking pan.
13. Sprinkle dried tart cherries on top.
14. Refrigerate for 30 minutes to set.
15. Cut into small clusters.

Storage: Keep in an airtight container in the refrigerator for up to 1 week.

Spirulina Recovery Bars

Ingredients:
- 1 cup dates
- 1/2 cup almonds
- 2 tablespoons spirulina powder
- 1/4 teaspoon Himalayan pink salt
- 2 tablespoons coconut oil
- 1 tablespoon raw cacao powder
- Chia seeds for topping

Instructions:
1. Remove pits from dates if necessary.
2. Place dates and almonds in a food processor and pulse for 2-3 minutes until mixture becomes a sticky, uniform dough.
3. Add spirulina powder to the food processor, pulsing 5-6 times to ensure even distribution of powder.
4. Sprinkle Himalayan pink salt over the mixture.
5. Melt the coconut oil in the microwave for 15 seconds.
6. Pour melted coconut oil into the food processor.
7. Pulse until ingredients are fully combined.
8. Line an 8x8-inch pan with parchment paper.
9. Transfer the mixture to the pan and press firmly to create an even layer.
10. Sprinkle raw cacao powder and chia seeds over the top.
11. Refrigerate for 1 hour until firm.
12. Lift out of the pan using parchment paper and cut into bars.

Storage: Refrigerate in an airtight container for up to 1 week.

Beet Root Bites

Ingredients:
- 1 cup raw cashews

Instructions:
1. Wash cucumber, apple, and parsley thoroughly.
2. Chop the cucumber and apple into small pieces.
3. Add cucumber, apple, and parsley to the blender.
4. Squeeze fresh lemon juice into the blender.
5. Sprinkle Himalayan pink salt over ingredients.
6. Grate a small piece of ginger (if using) into the mixture.
7. Add cold water and ice cubes.
8. Blend on high for 45-60 seconds until smooth.
9. Pour into a glass and serve immediately.

Storage: Best consumed fresh, will keep refrigerated for 2-4 hours.

Tropical Slim Surge

Ingredients:
- 1/2 cup papaya
- 1/2 cup pineapple
- 1/4 cup coconut water
- 1/4 cup spinach
- 1/4 teaspoon Himalayan pink salt
- 1/2 lime, juiced
- 3-4 ice cubes

Instructions:
1. Wash spinach thoroughly.
2. Peel and chop the papaya and pineapple into small pieces.
3. Add papaya, pineapple, and spinach to the blender.
4. Squeeze fresh lime juice into the blender.
5. Sprinkle Himalayan pink salt over ingredients.
6. Pour in coconut water.
7. Add ice cubes.
8. Blend on high for 45-60 seconds until smooth.
9. Pour into a glass and serve immediately.

Storage: Best consumed fresh, will keep refrigerated for 2-4 hours.

Spinach Hydration Elixir

Ingredients:
- 1 cup fresh spinach
- 1/2 green apple
- 1/2 cucumber

- 1/4 cup fresh mint leaves
- 1/4 teaspoon Himalayan pink salt
- 1/2 lemon, juiced
- 1/2 cup water
- 3-4 ice cubes

Instructions:
1. Wash spinach, apple, cucumber, and mint thoroughly.
2. Chop green apple and cucumber into small pieces.
3. Add spinach, apple, cucumber, and mint to the blender.
4. Squeeze fresh lemon juice into the blender.
5. Sprinkle Himalayan pink salt over ingredients.
6. Add water and ice cubes.
7. Blend on high for 45-60 seconds until smooth.
8. Pour into a glass and serve immediately.

Storage: Best consumed fresh, will keep refrigerated for 2-4 hours.

Watermelon Mineral Blast

Ingredients:
- 1 cup fresh watermelon
- 1/4 cucumber
- 1/4 cup fresh mint leaves
- 1/4 teaspoon Himalayan pink salt
- 1/2 lime, juiced
- 1/2 cup water
- 3-4 ice cubes

Instructions:
1. Wash the cucumber and mint thoroughly.
2. Cut watermelon into small cubes.
3. Chop the cucumber into small pieces.
4. Add watermelon, cucumber, and mint to the blender.
5. Squeeze fresh lime juice into the blender.
6. Sprinkle Himalayan pink salt over ingredients.
7. Add water and ice cubes.
8. Blend on high for 45-60 seconds until smooth.
9. Pour into a glass and serve immediately.

Storage: Best consumed fresh, will keep refrigerated for 2-4 hours.

Strawberry Recovery Smoothie

Ingredients:
- 1 cup fresh strawberries
- 1/2 cup unsweetened almond milk
- 1/4 cup spinach
- 1/4 teaspoon Himalayan pink salt
- 1/2 lemon, juiced
- 3-4 ice cubes
- Small piece of fresh ginger

Instructions:
1. Wash strawberries and spinach thoroughly.
2. Hull and chop strawberries into smaller pieces.
3. Add strawberries and spinach to the blender.
4. Squeeze fresh lemon juice into the blender.
5. Grate a small piece of ginger into the mixture.
6. Sprinkle Himalayan pink salt over ingredients.
7. Pour in unsweetened almond milk.
8. Add ice cubes.
9. Blend on high for 45-60 seconds until smooth.
10. Pour into a glass and serve immediately.

Storage: Best consumed fresh, will keep refrigerated for 2-4 hours.

Kale Detox Energizer

Ingredients:
- 1 cup fresh kale
- 1/2 green apple
- 1/2 cucumber
- 1/4 cup fresh parsley
- 1/4 teaspoon Himalayan pink salt
- 1/2 lemon, juiced
- 1/2 cup water
- 3-4 ice cubes

Instructions:
1. Wash kale, apple, cucumber, and parsley thoroughly.
2. Remove kale stems and chop into smaller pieces.
3. Chop green apple and cucumber.
4. Add kale, apple, cucumber, and parsley to the blender.
5. Squeeze fresh lemon juice into the blender.

6. Sprinkle Himalayan pink salt over ingredients.
7. Add water and ice cubes.
8. Blend on high for 45-60 seconds until smooth.
9. Pour into a glass and serve immediately.

Storage: Best consumed fresh, will keep refrigerated for 2-4 hours.

Citrus Lean Boost

Ingredients:
- 1/2 orange
- 1/2 grapefruit
- 1/4 cucumber
- 1/4 cup fresh mint leaves
- 1/4 teaspoon Himalayan pink salt
- 1/2 lime, juiced
- 1/2 cup water
- 3-4 ice cubes

Instructions:
1. Wash the cucumber and mint thoroughly.
2. Peel orange and grapefruit, removing all white pith.
3. Chop the orange, grapefruit, and cucumber into small pieces.
4. Add citrus fruits, cucumber, and mint to the blender.
5. Squeeze fresh lime juice into the blender.
6. Sprinkle Himalayan pink salt over ingredients.
7. Add water and ice cubes.
8. Blend on high for 45-60 seconds until smooth.
9. Pour into a glass and serve immediately.

Storage: Best consumed fresh, will keep refrigerated for 2-4 hours.

Apple Crisp Wellness Blend

Ingredients:
- 1 green apple
- 1/2 cup unsweetened almond milk
- 1/4 cup spinach
- 1/2 teaspoon cinnamon
- 1/4 teaspoon Himalayan pink salt
- 1/2 lemon, juiced
- 3-4 ice cubes
- Small piece of fresh ginger

- Optional: 1 tablespoon chia seeds

Instructions:
1. Wash the apple and spinach thoroughly.
2. Core and chop the apple into small pieces.
3. Add apple and spinach to the blender.
4. Squeeze fresh lemon juice into the blender.
5. Grate a small piece of ginger into the mixture.
6. Sprinkle Himalayan pink salt and cinnamon over ingredients.
7. Pour in unsweetened almond milk.
8. Add ice cubes and chia seeds (if using).
9. Blend on high for 45-60 seconds until smooth.
10. Pour into a glass and serve immediately.

Storage: Best consumed fresh, will keep refrigerated for 2-4 hours.

On-the-Go Tips

Between work deadlines, family obligations, and a never-ending to-do list, you need solutions that work in your real world, not just in some fantasy where you have unlimited time to prepare perfect meals. Here's how to get ahead of things with your Pink Salt Trick

Prep Like a Pro

Your Sunday night self determines your weekday success! Dedicate just 30 minutes each weekend to prep portable pink salt snacks that will save your butt all week long. Make double batches and store them in silicone reusable bags in the fridge. Portion everything into grab-and-go options.

Pink Salt Travel Kit

Create a mini pink salt emergency kit for your purse, desk drawer, or car! Fill a small container with a blend of pink salt, dried herbs, and lemon zest for an instant flavor boost that turns bland restaurant or cafeteria food into something that actually supports your goals. Pack a tiny jar with the Pink Salt Spice Blend so you're never stuck with bloat-inducing regular salt when dining out.

Smart Storage Solutions

Those beautiful mason jars might look social media-worthy, but they're not practical when you're running from meeting to meeting! Invest in leak-proof, BPA-free containers that actually fit in your bag without spilling everywhere. Silicone collapsible containers are perfect for Pink Salt Trail Mix, while small stainless steel containers work great for Pink Salt Chocolate Bites when you need that afternoon pick-me-up!

Sync With Your Morning Ritual

These on-the-go snacks work best when paired with your morning Pink Salt Trick! The minerals in your morning drink prime your cells for better absorption and utilization of nutrients throughout the day. When you follow up with strategic pink salt snacks, you're essentially reinforcing those metabolic benefits every few hours, keeping cravings at bay and energy stable from morning till night.

Travel Smart

Airports and road trips are food disaster zones! Pack TSA-friendly pink salt snacks like the Pink Salt Nut Mix in your carry-on (dry items pass security with no issues). For road trips, freeze your Pink Salt Lemonade in reusable bottles the night before—they'll thaw gradually as you travel, keeping your drink cold without diluting it with melting ice.

Hydration Amplifier

Those Pink Salt Spritzers aren't just delicious, they're portable hydration boosters! Fill a reusable water bottle with filtered water and add a tiny pinch of pink salt before heading out for the day. This simple hack helps your body actually retain the water you're drinking instead of just running straight to the bathroom every 30 minutes. This is especially crucial during workouts or on hot days!

Remember, consistency beats perfection every single time. Having one perfectly prepared pink salt meal at home isn't nearly as effective as incorporating moderate amounts of pink salt throughout your entire day, especially during those high-stress, high-temptation moments when your willpower typically caves.

Chapter 5:
Morning Rituals and Holistic Well-Being Using the Pink Salt Trick

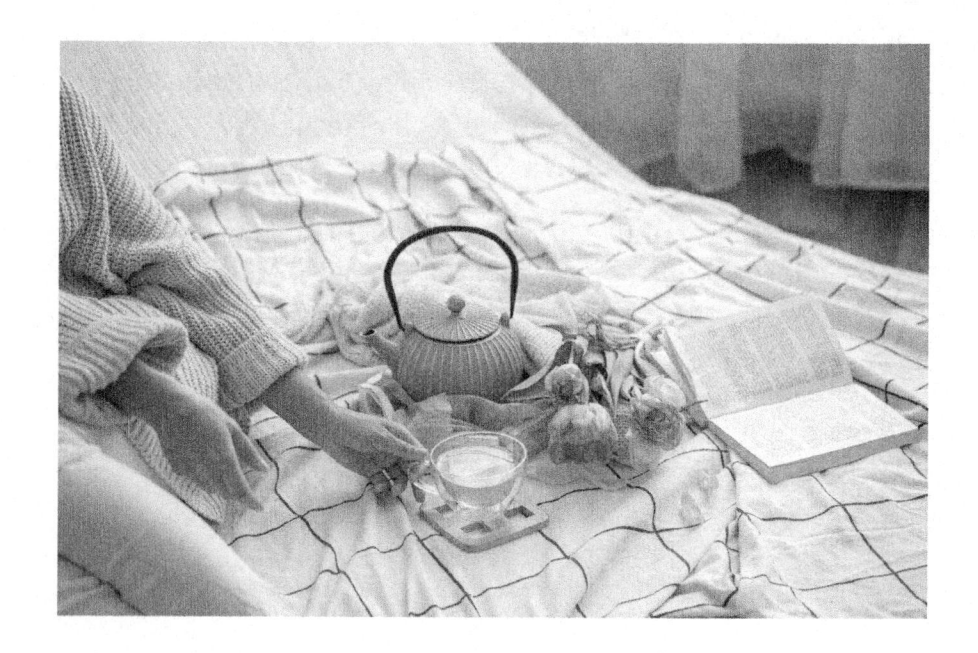

YOUR MORNING SETS the tone for everything that follows. Those first precious moments after you open your eyes are literally programming your body and mind for the next 16+ hours. Are you handing that power over to your smartphone and social media? Or are you claiming those moments for your health and well-being?

The Pink Salt Trick, as effective as it is, can't help your body lose weight and manage cortisol if you're not choosing to become mindful of your choices. Drinking your Pink Salt Trick masterpieces is now going to become the anchor of a transformative morning ritual that can completely overhaul how you look, feel, and function throughout your entire day.

Your morning ritual will become where the magic happens: when you expand this simple practice into a holistic approach to wellness that nourishes your body, mind, and spirit all at once.

Before you continue with this chapter, I want to make it clear that this isn't about adding complicated, time-consuming practices to your already-busy life. Instead of advocating for an intricate, hour-long routine, we're focusing on time-efficient, grounding activities that set me up for a happy and healthy day, no matter the season. These simple yet powerful rituals can be adapted to fit even the most hectic schedule, proving that you don't need hours of free time to transform your health.

Morning Pink Salt Rituals

Have you ever wondered why some mornings your body feels like it's working with you instead of against you? The reason for this is that timing is everything, especially when it comes to jumpstarting your metabolism after the overnight fast your body naturally experiences during sleep. The absolute metabolic sweet spot for your Pink Salt Trick is within 15 to 30 minutes of waking up, before consuming anything else.

Here is why this timing is so important. During sleep, your body becomes slightly dehydrated, and your cortisol naturally rises to help you wake up. That rising cortisol is your body's built-in mechanism for preparing to burn fat! But here's what most people get wrong: they immediately sabotage this natural fat-burning window by:

1. Reaching for caffeine first (which spikes cortisol even higher, creating stress that signals your body to hold onto fat).
2. Grabbing a carb-heavy breakfast (which shifts your body from fat-burning to glucose-burning instantly).
3. Checking email or social media (triggering stress responses that shut down metabolism).

Instead, when you consume your Pink Salt Trick during this critical morning window, you're providing your body with exactly what it needs to optimize that natural cortisol curve. The minerals in pink salt help regulate your fluid balance, support adrenal function, and prepare your digestive system to efficiently process nutrients throughout the day.

The 5-Minute Mindfulness Multiplier

Most people completely underestimate how much their thoughts impact their physical health. Research shows that stress hormones like cortisol can trigger your body to store fat, especially around your midsection. Even more fascinating, these stress responses happen regardless of whether the stress is real (like running from danger) or perceived (like worrying about your day).

Mindfulness is a powerful, yet simple practice, that allows you to calm the stress response, making it your secret weapon against cortisol and fat accumulation. Pairing your Pink Salt Trick with even just 5 minutes of mindfulness practice hydrates your body and changes your hormonal environment to one that supports fat loss instead of fat storage.

Try this powerful morning ritual:

1. Prepare your Pink Salt Trick (recipe from Chapter 3).
2. Find a comfortable seated position, preferably near natural light.
3. Take three deep, diaphragmatic breaths (inhale for 4 counts, hold for 1, exhale for 6).
4. As you sip your Pink Salt drink, focus completely on the sensation: the temperature, the subtle mineral taste, how it feels traveling down your throat.

5. Between sips, place one hand on your heart and one on your belly.
6. Silently repeat this affirmation: "My body knows exactly how to return to balance. I trust its wisdom completely."

What makes this practice so powerful is that it triggers your parasympathetic nervous system, your body's "rest and digest" mode, which is the physiological state where healing, repair, and yes, fat metabolism, function optimally. When you drink your Pink Salt Trick mindfully, those minerals are being absorbed into a body that's primed to use them, rather than a stressed system that's just trying to survive.

The Gratitude-Salt Connection

If you think gratitude is just some fluffy, feel-good practice, think again. There's a fascinating physiological connection between expressing gratitude and how your body processes nutrients, including the minerals in your Pink Salt Trick.

When you consciously focus on gratitude, your body releases dopamine and serotonin, neurotransmitters that not only make you feel good but also play crucial roles in digestion, metabolism, and even how your cells respond to insulin. This creates a powerful synergy with the Pink Salt Trick because these positive neurochemicals enhance your body's ability to absorb and utilize the minerals you're consuming.

Here's a simple but transformative practice to pair with your morning Pink Salt Trick:

1. Before taking your first sip, hold your drink at heart level.
2. Close your eyes and bring to mind three specific things you're grateful for today (being specific is key—not just "my family" but "the way my daughter laughed at breakfast yesterday").
3. With each thing you name, visualize that gratitude filling your drink with healing light energy.
4. As you sip your Pink Salt Trick, imagine those minerals carrying your gratitude to every cell in your body.

This might sound simplistic, but the science behind this practice is rock solid. Studies have shown that positive emotional states actually improve digestive enzyme secretion and nutrient absorption. By pairing gratitude with your Pink Salt Trick, you're creating an optimal internal environment for those minerals to do their magic.

The 2-Minute Movement Miracle

Your lymphatic system, your body's natural detoxification highway, doesn't have its pump. It relies on physical movement to move fluid through your system and carry away waste products. This is why incorporating even just 2 minutes of strategic movement with your Pink Salt Trick can dramatically enhance its effects.

While your body is absorbing those precious minerals from your morning drink, add these simple movements to amplify their impact:

1. **Gentle Twist & Release:** Sitting comfortably, place your right hand on your left knee and your left hand behind you. Inhale to lengthen your spine, then exhale as you gently twist to the left. Hold for 3 breaths, then switch sides. This wrings out your internal organs like a sponge, helping release toxins.
2. **Lymphatic Bounce:** Stand with feet hip-width apart, knees slightly bent. Gently bounce up and down on your toes for 30 seconds. This movement activates your lymphatic system throughout your entire body, improving circulation of those pink salt minerals.
3. **Heart-Opening Breath:** Standing or sitting, interlace your fingers behind your back. Inhale as you gently lift your chest and gaze upward, exhale as you release. Repeat 5 times. This opens up the chest area where major lymph nodes are concentrated.

These movements aren't going to burn massive amounts of calories, but they do optimize how your body processes the Pink Salt Trick you just consumed. The gentle compression and release created by these movements help your lymph system flush out metabolic waste while simultaneously improving circulation of those beneficial minerals throughout your body.

When it comes to transformative morning rituals, consistency trumps intensity every time. These simple practices take minutes, not hours, but their cumulative effect on your metabolism, hormones, and overall well-being is truly remarkable. Your body is waiting for these signals to optimize its natural functions. Give it what it needs, and watch how quickly it responds.

Evening Salt Routines

You've mastered the morning ritual, but what about those tricky evening hours when cravings hit hardest and your willpower is at its lowest? Evening routines with pink salt aren't just about relaxation (though they definitely help with that); they're strategic tools for conquering the most common diet saboteurs that show up after sunset.

The Craving Crusher

Many of us don't understand what truly happens between 8 PM and 9 PM when those intense cravings for sweet, salty, or carb-heavy foods seem to appear out of nowhere. These aren't a sign of weak willpower, they're your body's response to mineral imbalances and dehydration that have accumulated throughout your day.

A simple pink salt trick drink, Sole Water, at night time works one way in the morning, but completely differently during the evenings.

Sip this slowly, about 90 minutes before bedtime, while doing something relaxing, not while scrolling on your phone or watching intense TV shows. This timing is crucial because research suggests that a healthy salt intake may improve your sleep patterns and combat disturbed sleep (M. Zelman, 2024).

The science behind this is fascinating. Many nighttime cravings are actually mineral deficiencies in disguise. Your body knows it needs magnesium or potassium, but it doesn't know how to ask for them directly, so it triggers cravings for foods that might contain those minerals (along with loads of sugar, fat, and calories). By giving your body the pure minerals it's seeking, you short-circuit those misleading cravings!

Tension-Melting Salt Rituals

After a long, stressful day, your body is likely swimming in cortisol. Pink salt doesn't only work when consumed. From body scrubs to relaxing baths and foot soaks, pink salt can signal your body and mind to relax and enter into a state of rest or digest.

Make sure to take a look at Chapter 8 for 10 luxurious pink salt recipes that can be incorporated into your evening routine (without drying out your skin).

While soaking your body or feet, or standing under a shower stream, visualize the day's stress dissolving into the water. This isn't just a mental exercise; it's creating a physical response in your body. The magnesium in pink salt helps relax tense muscles, while the warm water improves circulation to areas that may have become stagnant from sitting all day.

The magic happens on multiple levels: first, the pink salt helps draw toxins out through your skin. Second, the minerals in the salt are actually absorbed through your skin, supporting cellular function and hydration. And third, the relaxation response triggered by this ritual helps release pent-up emotions, allowing you to let go of past baggage and emotional burdens.

Gentle Evening Movement Synergy

Intense exercise before bed can disrupt sleep, but gentle movement paired with your Pink Salt Trick creates a powerful synergy for overnight fat metabolism. The key is choosing the right type of movement that supports, rather than hinders, your body's transition to sleep.

Try this simple evening ritual:

1. Drink half of your Evening Pink Salt Elixir.
2. Take a 10-minute gentle walk outside (or around your home if it's dark).
3. Complete 5 minutes of relaxing stretches focused on opening your hips and shoulders.
4. Finish the remainder of your Pink Salt Elixir.

This sequence helps circulate the minerals from your pink salt drink throughout your body, reduces cortisol levels, and activates your parasympathetic nervous system so that your body can focus on repair and recovery.

Wellness experts suggest that this approach works because after fasting overnight, your body is more responsive to minerals and can better utilize them for metabolic support. By giving your body this mineral boost before sleep, you're providing the raw materials needed for overnight repair and metabolic processes.

The walking component is especially important, as it helps escort glucose into your muscles rather than having it float around in your bloodstream where it might be stored as fat. Even just 10 minutes makes a dramatic difference in how your body processes nutrients overnight!

These evening routines aren't separate from your morning Pink Salt Trick; they're part of a complete daily rhythm that supports your metabolism around the clock. The real transformation happens when you create this full-circle approach that works with your body's natural cycles rather than against them!

Mindfulness Practices

Did you know that your mental state can flip a switch in your body that determines whether you store or burn fat? This connection has been known to French women for centuries, but the rest of the world is only just recently catching up. The connection between your thoughts and your metabolism is one of the most powerful yet overlooked factors in weight loss.

Daily Meditation

While many people think of meditation as something reserved for spiritual gurus sitting cross-legged for hours, the reality is that even brief meditation sessions can dramatically enhance how your body processes the minerals in your Pink Salt Trick. Research has revealed a fascinating connection between meditative states and improved nutrient absorption.

A 2023 study found that people who combined mindfulness practices with their weight loss efforts experienced an average weight loss of 9 pounds compared to those using traditional approaches alone (Richards, 2023). This isn't just a coincidence, meditation creates physiological changes that support metabolism.

Try this simple 3-minute meditation after consuming your Pink Salt Trick:

1. Sit comfortably with your spine straight but not rigid
2. Place your palms on your knees, facing upward to symbolize openness to receiving
3. Close your eyes and bring awareness to where you can feel the Pink Salt Trick traveling through your body
4. With each inhale, imagine the minerals being distributed to every cell
5. With each exhale, visualize your body releasing what no longer serves it
6. After 3 minutes, open your eyes and take a moment to notice how you feel

Research has shown that mindfulness practices can alter amygdala functional connectivity, which plays a crucial role in maintaining weight loss rather than just achieving it temporarily.

Body Scanning for Deeper Awareness

One powerful mindfulness practice that works beautifully with the Pink Salt Trick is the body scan. This is a systematic method of bringing awareness to different parts of your body without judgment.

This practice helps break the disconnection many of us feel from our physical selves, which often leads to mindless eating and ignoring hunger/fullness cues.

Health experts recommend taking a few moments each day to scan your body from head to toe, observing any physical sensations or tension, to build a deeper mind-body connection that allows you to identify stress and emotional triggers before they lead to unhealthy eating patterns.

Here's how to practice a simple body scan while the minerals from your Pink Salt Trick circulate:

1. Lie down or sit comfortably with your eyes closed
2. Begin by bringing awareness to your feet, noticing any sensations without trying to change them
3. Slowly move your attention upward through your legs, hips, abdomen, chest, hands, arms, shoulders, neck, and head
4. As you scan, notice areas where you might be holding tension or stress
5. When you reach areas of tension, imagine the minerals from your Pink Salt Trick flowing there, bringing relaxation and healing.
6. Complete the scan by taking a moment to feel your entire body as a whole

This practice helps you recognize the early warning signs of stress before they trigger unhealthy eating patterns.

Calming Yoga Flows to Enhance Mineral Absorption

The postures you choose can enhance how effectively your body absorbs and utilizes the minerals in your Pink Salt Trick! Gentle, flowing movements help improve circulation, reduce cortisol, and optimize lymphatic drainage, all of which support your body's ability to use those precious minerals for metabolic processes rather than storing them as water weight.

Try this simple 5-minute sequence after your Pink Salt Trick:

1. **Mountain Pose with Deep Breathing:** Stand tall, feet hip-width apart. Inhale deeply through your nose as you raise your arms overhead, exhale completely as you lower them. Repeat 5 times to activate your parasympathetic nervous system.
2. **Gentle Twists:** Sitting or standing, place your right hand on your left knee and your left hand behind you. Inhale to lengthen your spine, exhale as you gently twist to the left. Hold for 3 breaths, then switch sides. This massage-like action for your internal organs helps stimulate digestion and mineral absorption.
3. **Forward Fold with Shoulder Release:** Stand with feet hip-width apart, knees slightly bent. Interlace your hands behind your back, then fold forward, allowing your clasped hands to fall forward over your head. This gentle inversion helps improve circulation throughout your body.
4. **Child's Pose:** Kneel on the floor, sit back on your heels, then fold forward with arms extended. This deeply calming pose signals your nervous system that it's safe to rest and digest, the perfect state for optimal nutrient absorption.

Basic Somatic Weight Loss Poses

Beyond traditional yoga, specific somatic poses (movements that connect mind and body awareness) can directly target areas where stubborn fat and emotional tension are stored. These poses aren't about forcing your body to change, they're about creating awareness and releasing the physical patterns that may be keeping you stuck.

Try these three powerful somatic movements:

1. **Belly Breathing Release:** Lie on your back with knees bent, feet flat on the floor. Place one hand on your belly and one on your heart. Inhale deeply through your nose, feeling your belly rise first, then your chest. Exhale completely through your mouth, drawing your navel toward your spine. Repeat 10 times, visualizing tension melting away from your midsection with each exhale.
2. **Hip Unwinding:** Still lying on your back, let your knees fall to one side while keeping both shoulders on the floor. Stay here for 5 deep breaths, noticing any tightness or holding patterns in your hips and lower back. Slowly return to center and repeat on the other side. Many people store emotional stress in their hips—this gentle release helps free both physical and emotional tension.
3. **Shoulder Meditation:** Sitting comfortably, slowly draw your shoulders up toward your ears on an inhale, then circle them back and down on the exhale, creating space across your collarbones. Repeat 5 times, then reverse direction. As you release your shoulders, imagine letting go of the burdens you've been carrying: perfectionism, self-criticism, and unrealistic expectations about your body.

Mindfulness practices don't need to be complicated or time-consuming to be effective. Even five minutes of intentional focus while sipping your Pink Salt Trick can create profound shifts in your stress levels, eating patterns, and ultimately, your body composition.

Start your Pink Salt Trick morning ritual and add an evening routine tonight to unlock holistic wellness. No more waiting for the "perfect time" to transform your health. That perfect moment is now. Your body has been patiently waiting for you to give it the mineral support it desperately needs, and every day you delay is another day spent fighting against your biology instead of working with it.

Chapter 6:
7-Day Pink Salt Trick Healing Challenge

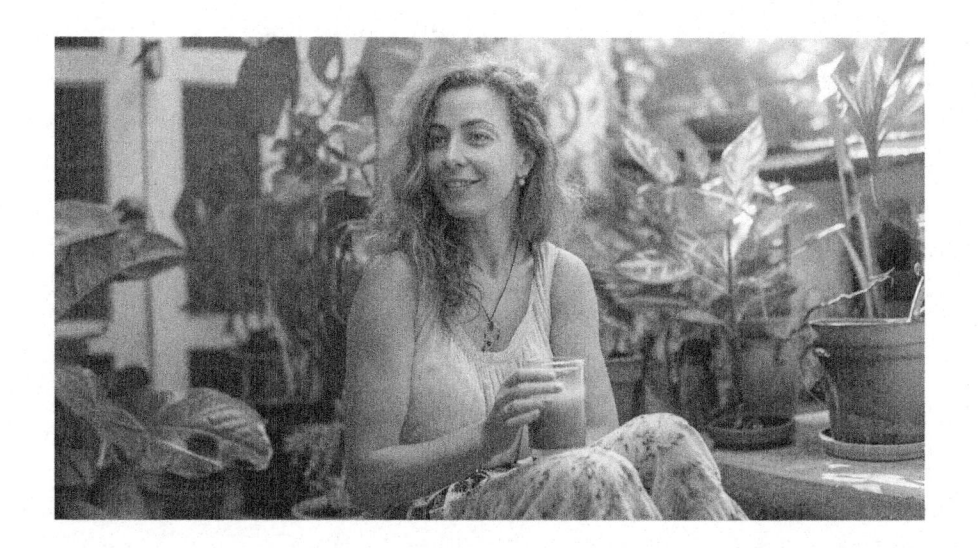

YOU'VE LEARNED THE science. You've got the recipes. You understand the "why" behind it all. But let's be honest, knowing something and doing something are two entirely different things!

That's exactly why I created the 7-Day Pink Salt Trick Healing Challenge for you. This is a strategic, sustainable approach that anyone can follow, even with a crazy schedule, picky family members, or minimal cooking skills.

Think of this week-long challenge as your metabolic reset button. After months (or years) of your body operating in survival mode, clinging to fat, fighting against your best efforts, leaving you exhausted and frustrated, this simple 7-day plan creates the perfect conditions for your system to finally release what it's been desperately holding onto.

What makes this challenge different from every other "quick fix" program you've tried? It works with your body's natural wisdom instead of forcing it into submission.

How the Challenge Works

The 7-Day Pink Salt Trick Healing Challenge isn't reinventing the wheel. All you're going to do is bring together everything you've learned so far into a streamlined, easy-to-follow system that creates dramatic results without dramatic effort. Think of it as your metabolic blueprint for the week, designed to remove all guesswork and decision fatigue.

The Daily Foundation
Each day of the challenge follows the same basic structure, creating consistency that your body craves:

1. **Morning Pink Salt Trick ritual:** You'll start each day with one of the Pink Salt Trick recipes from Chapter 3, consumed within 30 minutes of waking. This morning ritual kickstarts your metabolism, balances electrolytes, and sets the stage for proper hydration throughout the day.
2. **Strategic meal timing:** Rather than focusing on strict calorie counting or elimination diets, the challenge emphasizes when you eat certain foods, allowing your body's natural circadian rhythms to optimize digestion and fat-burning.
3. **Pink Salt-enhanced recipes:** You'll incorporate the delicious snacks and meals from Chapter 4 throughout your day, keeping your mineral levels balanced and your taste buds satisfied without triggering cravings or energy crashes.
4. **Evening wind-down ritual:** Each day concludes with one of the evening routines from Chapter 5, creating a full-circle approach that supports your body's natural detoxification and repair processes while you sleep.

The beauty of this structure is its simplicity. Once you understand the basic framework, you can adapt it to your preferences and lifestyle while still maintaining the core elements that drive results.

The Three Pillars of Transformation
While the day-to-day plan is incredibly straightforward, the challenge revolves around three key pillars that make it uniquely effective:

Deep Hydration (not just drinking water)
Most people think they're hydrated because they drink enough water, but without the proper mineral balance, much of that water passes right through without actually hydrating your cells. The challenge prioritizes "functional hydration," strategic consumption of mineral-rich fluids that your body can actually use.

This means sipping Pink Salt-infused water and herbal teas throughout the day, not just chugging plain water. The minerals act as transporters, helping fluid enter your cells where it's needed most. This cellular hydration is the foundation for all metabolic processes, including fat-burning.

Mindful awareness (not strict restrictions)
Instead of rigid rules about what you can't eat, the challenge focuses on building awareness around how different foods make you feel. You'll practice simple mindfulness techniques before meals and check in with your body afterward, gradually developing the ability to distinguish between true hunger and emotional eating.

This approach shifts you from the deprivation mindset of traditional diets to an abundance mindset. You're adding in nourishing foods and practices rather than focusing on what's forbidden. The result is sustainable change without the psychological backlash that derails most restrictive plans.

Gentle movement (not punishing workouts)
The challenge includes specific recommendations for light movement that enhance the effects of the Pink Salt Trick without overtaxing your system. These aren't calorie-torching HIIT sessions or marathon workouts. They're strategic, brief movement patterns designed to activate your lymphatic system, improve circulation, and enhance mineral absorption.

You'll incorporate simple movements that can be done in just minutes, regardless of your fitness level or available equipment. The focus is on consistency rather than intensity, allowing your body to heal and rebalance without the added stress of extreme exercise.

The progressive approach
What truly sets this challenge apart is how each day builds upon the previous one, creating a progressive journey rather than a static plan. The first few days focus heavily on establishing the foundational habits and allowing your body to adjust to its new mineral-rich environment. As the week continues, you'll gradually add more advanced practices and recipes, expanding your toolkit while maintaining the core rituals.

This progressive structure is specifically designed to prevent the overwhelming feeling that leads most people to abandon new health initiatives. Instead of changing everything at once, you'll make sustainable shifts that compound over the seven days, creating momentum that carries forward beyond the challenge itself.

By the end of the week, these practices won't feel like a "challenge" anymore. They'll feel like your new normal, a set of habits that support your body so effectively you won't want to go back to your old ways. That's the ultimate goal: not just seven days of results, but a foundation for lasting transformation.

7-Day Plan

Day	Morning Drink	Morning Movement	Midday Snack	Evening Drink	Evening Ritual
Day 1: Reset	Pink salt drink of your choice.	5-minute gentle stretching focusing on spine mobility.	Pink Salt snack.	Evening Pink Salt drink.	3-minute gratitude meditation before bed
Day 2: Hydrate	Pink salt drink of your choice.	10-minute walking (indoors or outdoors)	Pink Salt snack.	Evening Pink Salt drink.	5-minute body scan from toes to head
Day 3: Detoxify	Pink salt drink of your choice.	Lymphatic Bounce (30 seconds gentle bouncing, 3 sets)	Pink Salt snack.	Evening Pink Salt drink.	Pink salt foot soak while reading
Day 4: Balance	Pink salt drink of your choice.	5-minute yoga flow focusing on balance poses	Pink Salt snack.	Evening Pink Salt drink.	Bedtime journaling with 3 wins from the day

Day 5: Restore	Pink salt drink of your choice.	Heart-Opening Stretch Series (5 minutes of gentle chest openers)	Pink Salt snack.	Evening Pink Salt drink.	10-minute salt bath soak for feet or full body
Day 6: Energize	Pink salt drink of your choice.	Morning sun salutation (simplified, 5 repetitions)	Pink Salt snack.	Evening Pink Salt drink.	Evening stretching focused on the hips and shoulders
Day 7: Thrive	Pink salt drink of your choice.	15-minute nature walk (focus on deep breathing)	Pink Salt snack.	Evening Pink Salt drink.	Full 10-minute meditation on future health vision

Daily Focus Areas

Day 1: Reset
Today is about establishing your baseline and preparing your body for the week ahead. Keep everything simple and focus on consistency rather than perfection.

Day 2: Hydrate
Today emphasizes deep cellular hydration. Aim to drink half your body weight (in pounds) in ounces of water throughout the day, adding a pinch of pink salt to every other glass.

Day 3: Detoxify
Focus on supporting your body's natural detoxification pathways with extra movement and mineral support.

Day 4: Balance
Today is about finding equilibrium between activity and rest, savory and sweet, effort and ease.

Day 5: Restore
Prioritize self-care and restoration to support your body's healing processes.

Day 6: Energize
Build on the foundation you've created to tap into your body's natural vitality.

Day 7: Thrive
Celebrate your progress and set intentions for continuing these practices beyond the challenge.

Other Daily Guidelines
- **Hydration**: Drink at least 8 glasses of water throughout the day, adding a tiny pinch of pink salt to every other glass
- **Meals**: Focus on whole, unprocessed foods whenever possible, but no need for strict elimination
- **Timing**: Try to finish eating 3 hours before bedtime to support quality sleep

- **Awareness**: Notice how different foods affect your energy, mood, and digestion without judgment
- **Movement**: In addition to the suggested morning movements, take a 5-minute movement break for every 2 hours of sitting
- **Sleep**: Aim for 7-8 hours of quality sleep each night, keeping your bedroom cool and dark

This challenge is not about perfection, it's about progress. If you miss a step or modify something to fit your needs, simply continue with the next practice. The power is in the cumulative effect of these small, consistent actions rather than following the plan flawlessly.

Safety Guidelines

The Pink Salt Trick is generally safe for most people, but it's important to understand proper usage to get the benefits without overdoing it. Here are simple, practical guidelines to follow during your 7-Day Challenge:

For the Pink Salt Trick Challenge, follow these easy-to-remember guidelines:

- Morning ritual: Use ¼ teaspoon of pink Himalayan salt in your morning drink (about 1,150 mg of sodium)
- Evening ritual: Use ¼ teaspoon of pink Himalayan salt (about 575 mg of sodium)
- Throughout the day: Add no more than an additional ¼ teaspoon total to your water or food

This adds up to approximately a teaspoon daily, which provides minerals without exceeding healthy sodium limits. Health experts recommend keeping to 2,300 milligrams of daily sodium intake (about a teaspoon of salt total), including all sources in your diet.

The Hydration-Salt Balance

The most important safety guideline is maintaining proper hydration with your salt intake:

- **Water ratio**: Drink at least 8-10 ounces of water for every ¼ teaspoon of pink salt consumed
- **Daily minimum**: Aim for at least 64 ounces (8 cups) of water daily during the challenge
- **Timing**: Space out your salt and water intake throughout the day rather than consuming all at once

Who Should Modify or Avoid the Challenge

While the Pink Salt Trick is safe for most people, certain individuals should consult their healthcare provider before starting:

- People with high blood pressure or heart conditions
- Those with kidney disease or on potassium-restricted diets
- Individuals taking medications that interact with sodium
- Pregnant or nursing women
- Anyone with edema or fluid retention issues

If you experience headaches, excessive thirst, swelling, or dizziness during the challenge, reduce your pink salt intake immediately and increase water consumption.

The guidelines above work for most people, but individual needs vary based on factors like activity level, climate, and your unique physiology. Always pay attention to how your body responds and adjust accordingly. The Pink Salt Trick should leave you feeling energized and balanced, never bloated, thirsty, or uncomfortable. The goal isn't to consume as much pink salt as possible, it's to provide your body with just the right amount of minerals to support optimal function.

Tracking Progress

The true magic of the Pink Salt Trick Challenge is following the steps **and** noticing how your body responds. Tracking specific markers throughout your 7-day journey helps you stay motivated and also uncover personalized insights about what works specifically for your unique body.

Forget obsessing over just the number on the scale. The Pink Salt Trick works on multiple levels, so we need to track various indicators to capture your full transformation:

Daily Measurements
- **Morning weight:** Weigh yourself at the same time each morning after using the bathroom but before eating or drinking.
- **Water retention:** Note how your rings fit and whether your face or ankles appear puffy.
- **Measurements:** Take waist, hip, and thigh measurements before starting and on day 7 (measuring more frequently can lead to frustration as changes take time).

Subjective Tracking
- **Energy levels:** Rate your energy on a scale of 1-10 at three points daily: morning, afternoon, and evening.
- **Cravings intensity:** Note when cravings hit, what you're craving, and rate the intensity from 1-10.
- **Mood quality:** Track your overall emotional state using simple terms like "irritable," "calm," "motivated," or "anxious."
- **Sleep quality:** Each morning, rate last night's sleep from 1-10 and note how many times you woke up.

Physical Indicators
- **Digestion:** Track bowel movements (frequency and quality) as improved mineral balance often enhances digestive function.
- **Skin clarity:** Note changes in complexion, especially if you typically experience breakouts or dullness.
- **Mental clarity:** Record how easily you can focus and whether brain fog improves.

Progress Journaling

A simple daily journal can transform your Pink Salt Trick experience from a diet into a discovery. Here's how to create a journal that works:

The 2-minute check-in method

Each evening, take just two minutes to answer these three powerful questions:

1. What positive changes did I notice in my body today?
2. What was easier today than yesterday?
3. What will I do tomorrow to support my success?

This quick reflection reinforces positive changes, builds momentum, and creates a bridge to the next day's success. Your journal will reveal patterns you'd otherwise miss. Use these prompts to uncover them:

- "I notice my cravings intensify when..."
- "My energy seems highest after I..."
- "I feel most satisfied when..."

These patterns are **gold** because they reveal your body's unique responses and help you customize the Pink Salt Trick specifically for your needs.

Once you have these insights, you can create a simple chart with the days of the week across the top and your key metrics down the side. Use colors, symbols, or numbers to mark your daily progress. This visual representation helps you see improvements at a glance and provides a powerful motivational tool when you're tempted to skip a day.

Accountability Amplifiers

Tracking works even better with accountability. Here are some ways you can strengthen your commitment:

- Tell at least one supportive person about your 7-Day Pink Salt Trick Challenge. Research shows we're 65% more likely to complete a goal when we've told someone else about it.
- Take a quick selfie each morning (same lighting, same pose) to visually document subtle changes in skin, facial puffiness, and overall appearance. These visual cues can be incredibly motivating when written metrics don't seem to be changing.
- Find a friend to do the challenge with you, even long-distance. Send each other a quick daily text with your Pink Salt Trick victories for that day.

Don't wait until day 7 to acknowledge your progress. Create mini-celebrations for these milestone moments:

- First morning you wake up feeling less bloated.
- First time you notice your afternoon energy didn't crash.

- First sugar craving that you observed without acting on.
- First night of noticeably improved sleep.

These "little wins" compound into major transformations when properly acknowledged.

Kick off the 7-Day Pink Trick Healing Challenge today and watch your body and energy transform in just one month! The tools are in your hands. The plan is clear. The science is solid. Now it's time to take that crucial first step that separates those who wish for change from those who create it.

Your body has been waiting for this precise combination of minerals, mindfulness, and movement: the three pillars that work synergistically to unlock your natural fat-burning potential and restore vibrant energy. Unlike complicated programs that require massive lifestyle overhauls, this 7-day challenge slides effortlessly into your existing routine while delivering powerful results.

Chapter 7:
Weight Loss Management After the Challenge

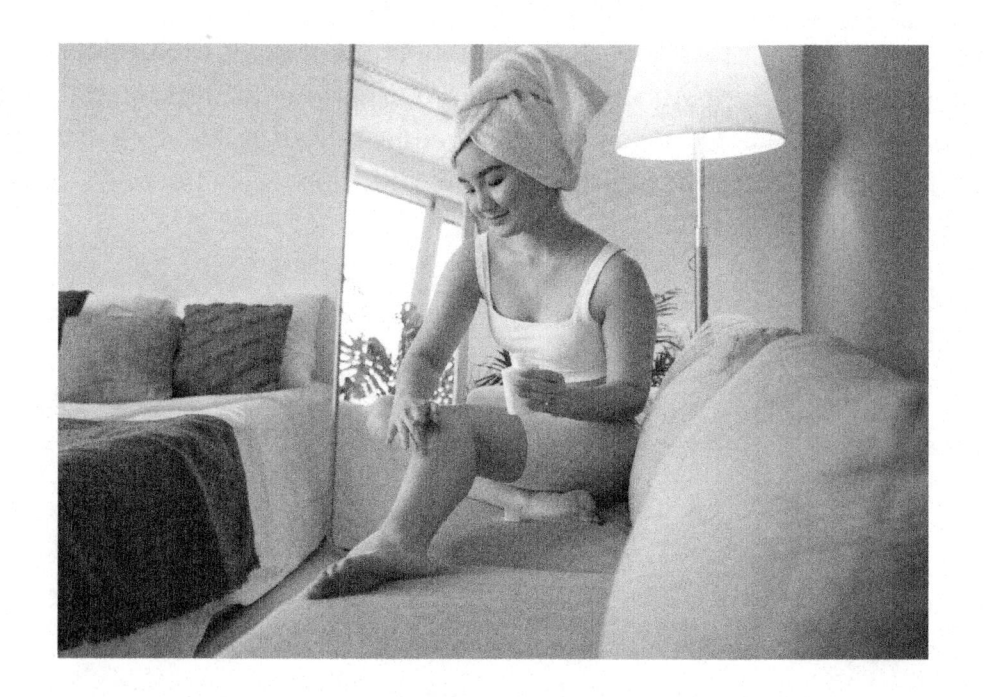

THE 7-DAY PINK SALT Trick Challenge is like lighting a match that creates an initial spark of change in your body. But the real magic happens when you transform that spark into a steady flame that burns bright long after the challenge ends. The truth about successful weight management isn't found in quick fixes or extreme measures. It's in the sustainable daily habits that silently reshape your metabolism, cravings, and energy day after day, year after year.

If you're like most people, you've probably experienced the frustration of losing weight only to gain it all back, plus a few extra pounds for good measure. You're not alone. Research reveals that only about 20% of people succeed at maintaining weight loss when it's defined as losing at least 10% of body weight and keeping it off for at least a year (Wing & Phelan, 2005). The good news is that you now possess something most people don't: a metabolic reset tool based on mineral balance rather than deprivation.

The Pink Salt Trick isn't a diet you "go on" and then "go off." It's a fundamental shift in how your body processes nutrients, balances fluids, and regulates the very hormones that control hunger, energy, and fat storage. By continuing these practices beyond the 7-day challenge, you're not just maintaining weight loss; you're creating lasting transformation at the cellular level.

Sustaining the Pink Salt Trick

The difference between people who maintain their weight loss and those who don't isn't willpower or genetics. It's consistency with the right habits! Research from the National Weight Control Registry shows that 94% of successful weight maintainers increased their physical activity and established consistent dietary patterns that they stuck with long-term (Hopkins Medicine, 2025). Your morning Pink Salt Trick ritual is the cornerstone habit that makes everything else easier!

Making your morning Pink Salt Trick a non-negotiable part of your daily routine, just like brushing your teeth, creates a metabolic foundation that supports everything else. It's the first decision you make each day that signals to your body, "We're taking care of business today!"

Here's how to cement this habit for the long haul:

1. **Prep the night before:** Keep a glass and your pink salt on your nightstand or bathroom counter where you'll see it first thing. This tiny step eliminates decision fatigue when your willpower is naturally lowest. Or use one of our overnight prep recipes!
2. **Link it to an existing habit:** The habit-stacking technique is **powerful**! If you always shower in the morning, place your Pink Salt Trick supplies right by the shower so you can do it immediately after. Your brain forms stronger neural pathways when you connect new habits to established ones.
3. **Create a trigger statement:** As you drink your Pink Salt Trick each morning, repeat a specific phrase like "My metabolism is firing up right now" or "My body knows exactly how to use these minerals." This mental programming amplifies the physical benefits through the mind-body connection.
4. **Track your streak:** Use a simple wall calendar or app to mark each day you complete your morning ritual. Research shows that keeping a daily record in a written journal, app, or spreadsheet can help identify what situations trigger unhealthy habits and provide accountability that keeps you on track. The longer your streak, the more motivated you'll be to maintain it!
5. **Have a backup plan:** Travel, illness, or unexpected events will happen. Create a travel kit with individual pink salt packets or a tiny container of pink salt that goes wherever you do. Think ahead about potential disruptions and how you'll handle them.

What makes this morning ritual so powerful for long-term success is that it's incremental rather than all-or-nothing. Forget the outdated notion that you need to overhaul your entire life to see results! Scientists have discovered that weight maintenance-specific behavioral skills help put into perspective the inevitable lapses and relapses of any long-term engagement. If you miss a day, simply resume the next morning without the guilt spiral that derails most people's efforts.

Incorporating Recipes into Regular Meals

The 7-Day Challenge introduced you to amazing Pink Salt recipes, but the magic happens when these become your new normal rather than special diet food. You need to upgrade your everyday meals with simple swaps that keep your mineral balance optimized!

Try these strategies to seamlessly integrate Pink Salt Trick recipes into your regular routine:

1. **The 50% rule:** Replace half of the regular salt in **all** your favorite recipes with pink Himalayan salt. This simple swap maintains familiar flavors while providing mineral benefits. Over time, gradually increase the proportion until you've fully transitioned.
2. **Strategic meal prep:** Choose 2-3 Pink Salt Trick recipes from Chapter 4 to prepare in larger batches each week. Store in grab-and-go containers for those moments when hunger strikes and willpower wanes.
3. **Family-friendly fusion:** Rather than cooking separate meals for yourself and your family, modify favorite family recipes with Pink Salt Trick principles. Pink salt-seasoned chicken nuggets, pink salt taco seasoning, or pink salt popcorn are easy wins that everyone will love.
4. **Restaurant strategy:** Keep a tiny container of pink salt in your purse or pocket for dining out. Most restaurants use heavily processed salt that won't provide the mineral benefits you need. A quick sprinkle of your own pink salt transforms any meal.
5. **The flavor-boosting technique:** Pink salt actually enhances your taste buds' sensitivity, meaning you need **less** salt overall to satisfy your palate. Place a few grains directly on your tongue before eating, and you'll find yourself naturally using less salt while enjoying flavors more intensely.

Avoiding Weight Regain

Losing weight isn't the hard part. Keeping it off is where the real challenge begins! Did you know that without proper maintenance strategies, up to 85% of people regain lost weight within a year? But you're not going to be one of those statistics because you have something they don't: the Pink Salt Trick as your metabolic insurance policy!

Your body's chemistry has fundamentally changed during the 7-Day Challenge. Your metabolism is firing again, your electrolyte balance is optimized, and your cravings have quieted down. Now it's time to leverage these advantages with smart nutrition strategies:

When planning meals after the challenge, follow this simple formula: **protein + plant food + pink salt = sustained success.** Research shows that improved maintenance of weight loss occurs when balanced energy expenditure is combined with proper nutrition strategies that prevent hunger and metabolic adaptation.

Try these Pink Salt-enhanced protein combos:

- Eggs sprinkled with pink salt and wrapped in lettuce
- Chicken breast with pink salt dry rub and roasted vegetables

- Greek yogurt with berries and a tiny pinch of pink salt

This combination helps maintain muscle mass while keeping hunger at bay, but the added pink salt makes all the difference by supporting your electrolyte balance.

The 2-Plate Strategy
One of the easiest ways to maintain portion control without counting calories is the 2-plate method:

1. Use a salad-sized plate for your main meal
2. Use a separate small bowl for any starchy carbs

This natural portion control tactic prevents the unconscious overeating that happens when everything is piled on one large plate.

The 80/20 Mineral Balance
Maintaining weight loss should never be about deprivation. You need to create the right mineral environment for your metabolism to thrive. Follow this simple rule: 80% of your meals should include pink salt and whole foods, while 20% can be more flexible.

For those flexible meals, still use pink salt as your seasoning, but don't stress about food choices. This prevents the all-or-nothing mentality that leads to bingeing.

Light Movement for Maintenance
Forget the punishing workouts that leave you exhausted, hungry, and with soaring cortisol levels! The Pink Salt Trick, combined with strategic light movements, creates the perfect synergy for weight maintenance.

Get walking, aim for as many steps a day as you can. I know that health gurus say 10,000 steps a day, but that number is literally pulled out of nowhere! Any movement is good movement. Don't want to walk, buy a Hoola Hoop, or turn up the music and dance for 30 minutes in your living room every day.

Try to get outdoors for at least three exercise sessions a week. A little bit of sun and vitamin D goes a long way in helping to elevate your mood and strengthen your bones and muscles.

Yes, health experts do recommend 150 minutes of moderate exercise per week, but jumping right into this duration when you're sedentary is only going to stress your body out. Gradually build up your movement times, go gently on your body, and remember that incremental movement is better than no movement.

Finally, think about stretching at the end of every day. Even if you don't incorporate the exercises you learned earlier, try for 3 to 5 minutes of gentle stretching while focusing on deep breathing. This practice helps:

- Release tension that triggers stress eating
- Improve sleep quality (critical for weight maintenance)
- Enhance the overnight effects of your evening Pink Salt ritual

In the early phases of your weight loss journey, you're not exercising to burn calories. You're moving to enhance your body's metabolism and mineral utilization. This mindset shift removes the pressure to do intense workouts and makes movement something you look forward to!

The Pink Salt Trick Long-Term

As your body continues to receive the minerals it needs, you'll experience benefits that go far beyond what the scale shows.

- **Improved energy, digestion, and stress resilience:** When you continue using the Pink Salt Trick daily, you'll notice that your initial results not only stick around, they actually intensify.
- **Sustainable energy without crashes:** The balanced mineral intake from the Pink Salt Trick establishes a new normal for your energy levels. Unlike caffeine or sugar, which give you temporary highs followed by crashes, the minerals in pink salt support consistent cellular energy production all day long. Many people report that after 30+ days of the Pink Salt Trick, they spontaneously wake up earlier, feel mentally sharper throughout the day, and no longer experience the 3 PM slump that used to send them reaching for cookies or coffee.
- **Digestive transformation:** Your digestive system is where nutrient absorption happens, or doesn't happen. The minerals in pink salt support proper hydrochloric acid production in your stomach, enzyme activity in your small intestine, and beneficial bacteria in your colon. After several months of the Pink Salt Trick, many people notice: less bloating after meals, more regular bowel movements, reduced food sensitivities, and better absorption of nutrients from food. This improved digestion creates a virtuous cycle where better nutrient absorption leads to fewer cravings, which supports weight maintenance.
- **Next-level stress resilience:** One of the most remarkable long-term benefits of the Pink Salt Trick is how it transforms your body's response to stress. The minerals in pink salt support healthy adrenal function, which governs your stress response. Over time, this creates greater resilience to life's inevitable stressors. Instead of stress triggering cravings and emotional eating, your body maintains equilibrium. Many people report that situations that used to send them diving into a bag of chips no longer have the same effect.
- **Aging gracefully:** The minerals in pink salt play crucial roles in hundreds of cellular processes that affect how your body ages. From skin elasticity to bone density to cognitive function, these minerals provide the raw materials your body needs to maintain itself optimally. Many people notice improvements in skin appearance, hair quality, and even energy levels as the Pink Salt Trick becomes part of their daily life. These benefits often intensify over time as mineral reserves are replenished.
- **Hormonal harmony:** Whether you're dealing with PMS, perimenopause, or the daily fluctuations that affect both men and women, the minerals in pink salt support proper hormonal function. This can lead to more stable moods, better sleep quality, and even improved libido over time. The magnesium in pink salt is particularly important for hormonal balance, as it supports the liver's ability to metabolize excess estrogen and helps convert thyroid hormone to its active form.

- **Environmental protection:** We're exposed to countless environmental toxins daily, in our air, water, food, and personal care products. The minerals in pink salt help your body's natural detoxification systems function optimally, providing some protection against this constant onslaught. While no single strategy can completely shield you from environmental toxins, the Pink Salt Trick supports your liver, kidneys, and lymphatic system in their natural cleansing functions, creating greater resilience.

Making the Pink Salt Trick a non-negotiable part of your daily routine helps you maintain your current weight loss, **and** you're investing in your long-term health in ways that will continue to unfold and surprise you.

Overcoming Challenges

Even with something as game-changing as The Pink Salt Trick, life happens! Those chocolate cravings still knock at 3 PM, and sometimes your schedule gets so packed that meal prep feels like a foreign concept. But the solution is literally expecting less from yourself.

- **Ditch the diet mentality:** You don't need another punishing plan you'll abandon by day three. You need to become your body's best friend, not its biggest critic.
- **Celebrate non-scale victories:** I know I said it before, but our transformation begins long before the number on the scale budges. Notice how your afternoon energy soars, how your rings slip on more easily as inflammation fades, how your skin glows from the inside out. These daily wins fuel your commitment more powerfully than any number ever could.
- **Make peace with your perfect imperfection:** Women in their 30s, 40s, and beyond are often harder on themselves than anyone else. Missing a day of your pink salt ritual doesn't erase your progress! Eating one fast food burger isn't going to destroy your body, and choosing not to move because you're feeling less than energetic isn't going to put on 10 pounds. Your body is remarkably resilient; just pick up where you left off.

The Pink Salt Trick works because it addresses what your body is actually crying out for, deep cellular hydration and mineral balance. Your journey with the Pink Salt Trick doesn't end once you've reached your goals. This is about creating lasting change that transforms your relationship with your body for good. The beauty of this approach is its simplicity.

Don't forget to celebrate every victory, no matter how small. Each day you honor your body's needs is a win worth acknowledging.

Chapter 8:
The Pink Salt Trick for Lasting Well-Being

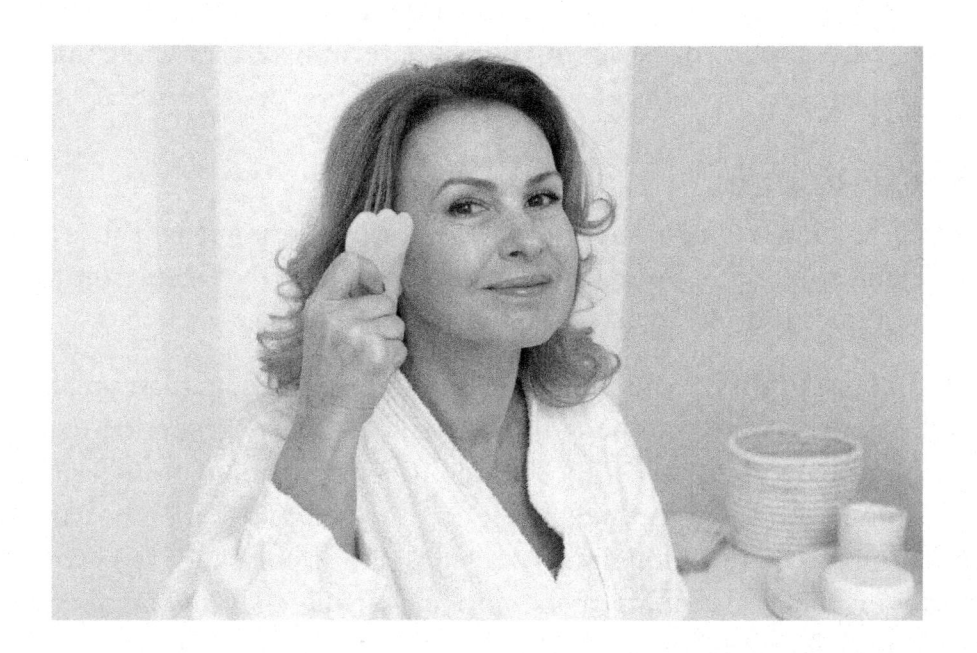

IMAGINE WAKING UP with skin that glows like you've had a $500 facial, muscles that recover from yesterday's workout with lightning speed, and energy levels that make your coworkers wonder what you've been drinking. This isn't fantasy, it's what happens when you take the miraculous minerals in pink salt beyond your morning hydration ritual and into every aspect of your wellness routine.

By now, you've experienced how the Pink Salt Trick transforms your metabolism and melts away stubborn pounds. We're just scratching the surface of what these ancient crystals can do for your total well-being. The same mineral-rich profile that balances your hormones and fires up fat burning also works magic on your skin, hair, recovery time, and even your emotional balance.

Beauty with Pink Salt

Pink Salt Body Scrub

Ingredients:
- 1/2 cup fine Himalayan pink salt
- 1/4 cup coconut oil
- 2 tablespoons sweet almond oil
- 5 drops of lavender essential oil

- 1 tablespoon dried rose petals

Instructions:
1. Melt coconut oil in the microwave for 15-20 seconds until liquid.
2. In a clean mixing bowl, combine Himalayan pink salt and melted coconut oil, stirring until fully integrated.
3. Add sweet almond oil and mix thoroughly to create a smooth consistency.
4. Gently add lavender essential oil, stirring to distribute evenly.
5. Fold in dried rose petals, ensuring they are well dispersed throughout the scrub.
6. Transfer mixture to a clean, dry glass jar with a tight-fitting lid.
7. Allow the scrub to cool and set at room temperature.

Storage: Store in a cool, dry place and use within 2 months.

Himalayan Salt Facial Mist

Ingredients:
- 1/2 cup distilled water
- 1 tablespoon Himalayan pink salt
- 2 tablespoons witch hazel
- 5 drops rose water
- 3 drops of vitamin E oil

Instructions:
1. Boil water and allow it to cool to room temperature.
2. In a clean glass bowl, dissolve Himalayan pink salt completely in water, stirring until no granules remain.
3. Add witch hazel to salt water and mix thoroughly.
4. Carefully add rose water, stirring gently to combine.
5. Incorporate vitamin E oil, mixing well.
6. Using a small funnel, transfer the mixture into a clean spray bottle.
7. Secure the bottle cap and shake well before each use.

Storage: Refrigerate and use within 1 month.

Mineral Glow Body Oil

Ingredients:
- 1/4 cup jojoba oil
- 2 tablespoons argan oil
- 1 tablespoon finely ground Himalayan pink salt
- 5 drops frankincense essential oil
- 3 drops of vitamin E oil
- Small dried calendula petals

Instructions:
1. In a clean glass bottle, combine jojoba and argan oils.
2. Using a mortar and pestle, grind Himalayan pink salt into fine powder.
3. Add ground salt to the oil mixture, shaking vigorously to distribute.
4. Add frankincense essential oil, ensuring even incorporation.
5. Drop in vitamin E oil as a natural preservative.
6. Sprinkle dried calendula petals into the bottle.
7. Seal the bottle and gently roll to mix ingredients.

Storage: Store in a cool, dark place. Use within 3 months.

Detox Salt Bath Soak

Ingredients:
- 1 cup Himalayan pink salt
- 1/2 cup Epsom salt
- 1/4 cup baking soda
- 2 tablespoons dried lavender
- 10 drops of eucalyptus essential oil

Instructions:
1. In a large mixing bowl, combine Himalayan pink salt and Epsom salt.
2. Sift baking soda over the salt mixture to prevent clumping.
3. Using clean hands, mix salts thoroughly.
4. Crush dried lavender between palms to release essential oils.
5. Sprinkle crushed lavender over the salt mixture.
6. Add eucalyptus essential oil, stirring to distribute evenly.
7. Transfer to a clean, dry glass jar with a tight-fitting lid.
8. Can be used as a foot soak as well.

Storage: Keep in a dry location, use within 6 months.

Overnight Skin Recovery Mask

Ingredients:
- 2 tablespoons honey
- 1 tablespoon Greek yogurt
- 1 teaspoon Himalayan pink salt
- 1 teaspoon aloe vera gel
- 3 drops rosehip oil

Instructions:
1. In a small mixing bowl, combine honey and Greek yogurt.
2. Sprinkle Himalayan pink salt over the mixture.

3. Stir until salt is completely dissolved.
4. Add aloe vera gel and mix thoroughly.
5. Carefully incorporate rosehip oil.
6. Whisk ingredients until smooth and uniform.
7. Apply a thin, even layer to clean skin before bedtime.
8. Leave on overnight and rinse with lukewarm water in the morning.

Storage: Prepare fresh for each use. Refrigerate the unused portion for 2-3 days.

Illness Recovery

Immune Defense Healing Broth

Ingredients:
- 4 cups bone broth
- 2 fresh shiitake mushrooms
- 1 inch fresh ginger root
- 2 cloves of garlic
- 1/4 teaspoon Himalayan pink salt
- 1 tablespoon fresh turmeric
- Small bunch of fresh thyme

Instructions:
1. Wash fresh shiitake mushrooms and pat dry.
2. Use a sharp knife to finely mince mushrooms into small, uniform pieces.
3. Using a microplane, grate ginger and turmeric root to release maximum flavor and nutrients.
4. Crush garlic cloves and let sit for 10 minutes to activate allicin compounds.
5. Place bone broth in a large pot and heat over medium flame.
6. Add minced mushrooms, grated ginger, turmeric, and crushed garlic to the broth.
7. Sprinkle Himalayan pink salt evenly across the surface of the broth.
8. Reduce heat and simmer gently for 15-20 minutes, allowing flavors to meld.
9. Remove from heat and strain through a fine-mesh strainer.
10. Serve warm in heat-safe mugs.

Storage: Refrigerate and consume within 48 hours.

Respiratory Relief Elixir

Ingredients:
- 1 cup hot water
- 1 tablespoon raw honey
- 1/2 lemon, juiced
- 1/4 teaspoon Himalayan pink salt

- 1 cinnamon stick
- 2 fresh thyme sprigs
- Small piece of fresh ginger

Instructions:
1. Boil water in kettle and let cool for 1-2 minutes to reach optimal brewing temperature.
2. Using a microplane, grate fresh ginger directly into a clean mug.
3. Pour hot water over grated ginger.
4. Cut the lemon in half and squeeze juice directly into the mug.
5. Add raw honey to the mug and stir until completely dissolved.
6. Sprinkle Himalayan pink salt evenly across the surface of the liquid.
7. Add a whole cinnamon stick and fresh thyme sprigs.
8. Let the mixture steep for 5-7 minutes, allowing herbs to infuse.
9. Remove herbs and cinnamon stick before drinking.
10. Stir once more and consume while warm.

Storage: Best consumed immediately, discard after 4 hours.

Fever Reduction Tisane

Ingredients:
- 1 cup elderberry tea
- 1 tablespoon fresh mint leaves
- 1/8 teaspoon Himalayan pink salt
- 1 tablespoon fresh lemon juice
- Small piece of fresh sage
- Optional: 1 teaspoon raw honey

Instructions:
1. Boil water and steep the elderberry tea bag for exactly 5 minutes.
2. Remove the tea bag and set aside.
3. Gently tear fresh mint and sage leaves by hand.
4. Add torn herbs directly to the steeped tea.
5. Sprinkle Himalayan pink salt evenly across the surface.
6. Cut the lemon in half and squeeze juice into the tea.
7. Optional: Drizzle raw honey and stir until incorporated.
8. Allow mixture to sit for 3 minutes to fully infuse herbs.
9. Strain through a fine-mesh strainer into a serving mug.
10. Serve warm.

Storage: Consume within 2 hours of preparation.

Gut Restorating Mineral Drink

Ingredients:
- 1 cup kefir
- 1/2 green apple
- 1 tablespoon fresh ginger
- 1/4 teaspoon Himalayan pink salt
- 1 tablespoon fresh parsley
- 1/2 cup water
- Optional: 1 tablespoon chia seeds

Instructions:
1. Wash the green apple and pat dry.
2. Core and chop the apple into small pieces.
3. Peel fresh ginger and grate using a microplane.
4. Chop fresh parsley into fine pieces.
5. Add kefir to the blender.
6. Add chopped apple and grated ginger.
7. Sprinkle Himalayan pink salt over the mixture.
8. Add water and fresh parsley.
9. Optional: Sprinkle chia seeds on top.
10. Blend on high for 45-60 seconds until smooth.
11. Pour into a glass and serve immediately.

Storage: Consume within 24 hours, refrigerate.

Inflammation Suppression Tonic

Ingredients:
- 1 cup fresh pineapple juice
- 1/2 teaspoon ground turmeric
- 1/4 teaspoon Himalayan pink salt
- 1 tablespoon fresh ginger
- 1/2 lemon, juiced
- Optional: 1 tablespoon raw honey

Instructions:
1. Juice the fresh pineapple or use pre-pressed juice.
2. Grate the fresh ginger using a microplane.
3. Pour pineapple juice into a glass.
4. Add ground turmeric and stir thoroughly.
5. Sprinkle Himalayan pink salt evenly.
6. Add grated ginger.

7. Squeeze fresh lemon juice.
8. Optional: Drizzle raw honey and mix well.
9. Stir until all ingredients are fully incorporated.
10. Serve at room temperature.

Storage: Consume immediately, discard after 2 hours.

Holistic Practices with Pink Salt

Are you ready to take your Pink Salt Trick to a whole new level of skin-glowing amazingness? You're not just here to drop a few pounds. You want to feel like your absolute best self from the inside out!

That's exactly why combining pink salt with ancient wellness practices is the beauty secret you've been desperately searching for. These aren't your grandmother's beauty routines (though she probably looked fabulous, too!). These are supercharged rituals that tackle those stubborn problem areas that creams and serums just can't touch. Let's get into it!

Face Yoga and Pink Salt Facial Mist

Your face has over 50 muscles that need just as much love as your body! Combining the mineral-packed Pink Salt Facial Mist with face yoga can yield incredible results, all without the $300 facelift bill or downtime!

Face yoga is a science-backed way to tone and tighten those forgotten facial muscles that gravity loves to pull downward after 35. When you pair specific facial movements with our Pink Salt Mist, you're essentially creating a workout-plus-hydration routine for your face that makes expensive creams look like child's play!

The magic happens because pink salt delivers trace minerals directly to your skin cells while you're actively increasing blood flow through targeted movements. Think about it: your cheekbones get an instant lift, those pesky forehead lines soften, and that jawline you thought disappeared years ago? She's coming back, honey!

Just 5 minutes each morning while spritzing our mineral mist will reawaken those sleeping facial muscles, flush out toxins that cause puffiness, and give you that "Did she get work done?" glow that lasts all day. Your makeup will glide on smoother, your confidence will soar, and the compliments? Get ready for them!

5-Minute Face Yoga Routine

These targeted movements instantly lift, tone, and revitalize tired facial muscles! Perform each exercise 10 times while applying your Pink Salt Facial Mist:

Cheekbone Sculptor:
1. Place your fingers at the center of your cheeks
2. Smile while pressing gently upward

3. Hold for 5 seconds, then release
4. Feel those forgotten muscles wake up as they get that mineral boost!

Forehead Smoother:
1. Place palms on forehead with fingers facing each other
2. Apply gentle pressure while sliding hands outward
3. The pink salt mist penetrates as you release tension lines!

Jawline Definer:
1. Tilt your head back slightly and look at the ceiling
2. Push the lower lip out as far as possible
3. Hold for 10 seconds while feeling the stretch
4. Your jawline will thank you for this mineral-infused workout!

Eye Rejuvenator:
1. Place index fingers at the outer corners of the eyes
2. Middle fingers at the inner corners
3. Gently press while squinting, then release
4. Say goodbye to crow's feet as those minerals work their magic!

For dramatic results, perform this routine daily after your morning Pink Salt Trick drink. Your face deserves the same mineral boost as the rest of your body!

Scalp Massage + Pink Salt Scalp Scrub

Your hair isn't just suffering from product buildup. It's mineral-starved! That's why combining a detoxifying Pink Salt Body Scrub with targeted acupressure points delivers incredible results that expensive salon treatments can't touch!

The secret lies in pink salt's ability to naturally exfoliate dead skin cells while balancing your scalp's pH and delivering essential trace minerals directly to your follicles. When paired with specific pressure points that increase circulation, you're essentially giving your hair roots a double-shot of revitalizing nourishment!

This treatment works wonders for thinning hair, excessive shedding, and that annoying itchy scalp that flares up during stressful weeks. The minerals in pink salt help regulate oil production, while the massage techniques release tension that's strangling your follicles from receiving proper nutrients.

Just 10 minutes once a week can transform lackluster locks into the thick, glossy hair you thought was only possible with expensive extensions! Plus, the stress-melting benefits of the acupressure points mean you'll walk away feeling like you've had a full-body massage. Hair growth and relaxation in one simple treatment? Yes, please!

Pink Salt Scalp Treatment

Ingredients:
- 2 tablespoons finely ground pink Himalayan salt
- 1 tablespoon coconut oil (warmed until liquid)
- 5 drops rosemary essential oil (proven to stimulate growth!)
- 3 drops peppermint essential oil (for circulation boost)
- Small bowl for mixing

3-Minute Hair Growth Acupressure Routine

These powerful pressure points activate your body's natural hair growth triggers while the minerals in your scalp treatment work their magic!

Crown Energizer:
1. Place your fingertips at the very top center of your head
2. Make small circular motions for 30 seconds
3. Feel the tingling? That's increased blood flow delivering those minerals!

Growth Activator Points:
1. Find the hollow areas behind your ears where your skull meets your neck
2. Press firmly for 10 seconds, release for 5 seconds
3. Repeat 3 times while taking deep breaths
4. These points connect directly to your hair's growth cycle!

Stress-Release Temple Press:
1. Place the index and middle fingers on the temples
2. Apply gentle pressure and rotate in small circles
3. Stress chokes your hair follicles. Feel it melting away!

For best results, use this treatment weekly as part of your Pink Salt beauty ritual. Your hair deserves the same mineral magic that's transforming the rest of your body!

Always rinse your hair thoroughly and follow up with a deep conditioner to prevent dryness.

Reflexology + Pink Salt Foot Soak

Your feet connect to every major organ in your body, yet they're the most neglected part of most beauty routines. Combining an energizing Pink Salt Foot Soak with targeted reflexology points creates an incredible detox pathway that affects everything from your digestion to your stress levels!

This treatment tackles multiple issues at once: swollen ankles, hormone imbalances, digestive troubles, and even those stubborn sleep problems. The minerals in pink salt help draw out toxins and reduce inflammation, while the reflexology points trigger your body's natural healing responses.

Just 15 minutes with this simple routine can leave you feeling lighter, more energized, and noticeably less bloated. For downloadable reflexology maps or tutorials, simply search online for "foot reflexology chart." There are countless free resources that show exactly which pressure points correspond to your trouble spots!

Pink Salt Foot Soak Recipe

This mineral-rich soak will transform tired feet while sending healing minerals throughout your entire body!

Ingredients:
- 1/2 cup Himalayan pink salt
- 1 tablespoon magnesium flakes (for extra relaxation)
- 3 drops lavender essential oil (sleep enhancer)
- 2 drops peppermint essential oil (energizing)
- Large basin or tub for soaking
- Warm water

Instructions:
1. Fill a basin with enough warm water to cover the ankles
2. Add pink salt and magnesium flakes
3. Add essential oils just before soaking
4. Swirl water to dissolve minerals completely

How to Use: Soak feet for 15-20 minutes while performing the reflexology routine below. For maximum benefit, pat feet dry without rinsing to allow minerals to continue absorbing overnight.

5-Minute Reflexology Routine

These powerful pressure points activate healing responses throughout your body while the minerals from your foot soak penetrate deeply!

Thyroid Balance Point:
1. Find the base of your big toe
2. Press firmly with your thumb for 30 seconds
3. Repeat on the other foot
4. Feel your metabolism getting that mineral boost!

Detox Liver Point:
1. Locate the soft area between your big toe and second toe
2. Apply firm pressure for 30 seconds
3. This helps your body process toxins more efficiently!

Digestive Relief Zone:
1. Find the center of your foot arch
2. Press and make small circles for 60 seconds

3. Perfect for reducing bloating and improving digestion!

Adrenal Balance Point:
1. Find the middle of your foot, right below the ball
2. Apply pressure and hold for 30 seconds
3. Helps regulate stress hormones while pink salt minerals work!

Use this treatment twice weekly as part of your Pink Salt beauty ritual for optimal results. Your tired feet deserve this mineral-rich spa treatment!

Tongue Scraping + Pink Salt Mouth Rinse

Did you know the white coating on your tongue each morning is toxins your body tried to expel overnight? This ancient Ayurvedic practice, paired with our mineral-rich Pink Salt Mouth Rinse, doesn't just freshen breath/ It's a complete digestive reset that impacts everything from your gut health to your skin clarity!

This powerful morning ritual works because tongue scraping physically removes accumulated toxins while the pink salt rinse delivers trace minerals directly to your oral microbiome. It's like giving your entire digestive system a fresh start every single day without expensive probiotics or complicated cleanses!

The benefits extend far beyond your mouth. This simple routine can diminish sugar cravings, improve nutrient absorption, boost immune function, and even help clear stubborn skin problems that stem from poor digestion. The minerals in pink salt help neutralize harmful bacteria while creating a balanced oral environment that supports your entire body.

Just 60 seconds each morning with this simple routine can dramatically shift your health trajectory and amplify the results of your Pink Salt Trick! Plus, you'll immediately notice fresher breath, clearer sinuses, and a cleaner mouth feeling that lasts all day. Who knew the secret to better digestion started on your tongue?

Pink Salt Mouth Rinse Recipe

This mineral-packed rinse delivers essential nutrients directly to your oral microbiome for whole-body benefits!

Ingredients:
- 1 cup filtered water
- 1/2 teaspoon Himalayan pink salt
- 1/4 teaspoon baking soda (optional for alkalizing)
- 2 drops food-grade peppermint oil (optional)
- Glass jar for storage

Instructions:
1. Heat water until warm but not boiling

2. Add pink salt and stir until completely dissolved
3. Add baking soda and peppermint oil if using
4. Allow to cool completely
5. Store in a sealed glass container for up to 5 days

How to Use: After tongue scraping, swish 2 tablespoons vigorously for 30 seconds, focusing on different areas of your mouth. For maximum detoxification benefits, do this before consuming any food or drink in the morning.

Morning Tongue Scraping Ritual

This simple detox technique removes accumulated toxins while preparing your body to absorb the minerals from your mouth rinse!

Step 1: Choose Your Scraper
1. Use a proper tongue scraper (copper or stainless steel works best)
2. Plastic scrapers or spoons don't remove toxins as effectively!

Step 2: Proper Technique
1. Stand in front of a mirror with your mouth open and tongue extended
2. Place the scraper at the back of the tongue (as far as comfortable)
3. Apply gentle pressure and pull forward to the tip of the tongue
4. Rinse the scraper after each pass
5. Repeat 3-5 times until no more residue appears
6. Those toxins you're removing were heading straight to your digestive system!

Step 3: Complete With Pink Salt Rinse
1. Immediately follow with your mineral-rich mouth rinse
2. Focus on swishing between teeth and along the gum line
3. Your clean tongue can now better absorb those essential minerals!

For best results, make this the very first thing you do each morning, even before drinking water. This allows you to remove overnight toxin buildup before it's reabsorbed into your system.

Acupressure + Pink Salt Compress

Those puffy eyes and tension headaches are your body's distress signals. Combining warm Pink Salt Compresses with targeted acupressure creates an incredible relief system that addresses both symptoms and their underlying causes in just minutes!

This powerful pairing works because the warm salt compress delivers mineral-rich heat directly to your tissues while acupressure points activate your body's natural healing pathways. It's like giving your lymphatic system and circulation a jump-start while simultaneously calming your nervous system!

The beauty benefits appear almost instantly: reduced under-eye bags, diminished facial puffiness, and noticeably relaxed expression lines.

Just 10 minutes with this simple routine can transform your appearance while melting away stress that accelerates aging. For the most effective acupressure points, simply search online for "facial acupressure points" or "acupressure for puffiness." You'll find numerous free diagrams showing exactly where to apply pressure for your specific concerns!

Pink Salt Compress Recipe

This mineral-rich compress delivers healing warmth and essential nutrients directly to your problem areas.

Ingredients:
- 1/4 cup Himalayan pink salt
- 1 cup water
- 1 tablespoon dried chamomile flowers (optional for extra soothing)
- Small cotton towel or washcloth
- Bowl for soaking

Instructions:
1. Heat water until hot but not boiling
2. Add pink salt and stir until completely dissolved
3. Add dried chamomile if using
4. Soak your cloth completely in the solution
5. Wring out until damp (not dripping)

How to Use: Apply a warm compress to each acupressure point for 30-60 seconds while applying gentle finger pressure. Reheat the compress as needed by dipping it back into the warm solution.

Quick Acupressure + Compress Routine

These powerful pressure points, paired with your mineral-rich compress, address common beauty concerns in minutes!

For Puffy Eyes:
1. Apply a warm compress to the entire eye area for 30 seconds
2. Find the indentation at the inner corner of each eyebrow
3. Press gently while applying the compress for another 30 seconds
4. Feel that stubborn morning puffiness melting away!

For Tension Headaches:
1. Place the compress at the base of your skull where your neck meets your head
2. Apply pressure with fingertips through the compress for 60 seconds
3. Feel the tension releasing as minerals penetrate deeply!

For Facial Bloating:
1. Apply a compress to just below your cheekbones
2. Press upward gently while holding the compress
3. Watch as your face regains its sculpted appearance!

For Jaw Tension:
1. Find the soft spot where your jaw hinges near your ears
2. Apply a warm compress with gentle circular pressure
3. Notice how your entire face relaxes as minerals soothe tight muscles!

For additional acupressure points tailored to your specific concerns, search online for "facial acupressure map" or watch tutorial videos. There are excellent free resources that show exactly which points address your particular beauty issues.

Use this treatment 2 to 3 times weekly as part of your Pink Salt beauty ritual, especially during high-stress periods or when you need to look your absolute best! Your face deserves this mineral-rich tension release!

Dry Brushing + Gua Sha with Pink Salt

Stubborn cellulite and morning puffiness are signs your lymphatic system is crying out for help! Combining Dry Brushing and Gua Sha with Pink Salt mineral treatments creates a powerful detox trio that transforms how your body processes fluids, toxins, and fat.

This revolutionary combination works because dry brushing manually stimulates lymph flow on larger body areas while gua sha provides targeted drainage on the face and neck. When paired with pink salt's mineral-rich properties, you're essentially creating a complete lymphatic reset that ordinary creams and serums simply can't touch!

The results are nothing short of dramatic: visibly reduced cellulite, diminished facial puffiness, clearer skin, and a noticeably more sculpted appearance overall. Plus, you'll experience improved energy levels as your body's natural detox pathways open up and begin functioning optimally again.

Just 5 minutes of dry brushing before your shower, followed by a quick facial gua sha routine with our mineral-infused oil, can completely transform how you look and feel.

Pink Salt Mineral Body Oil Recipe

This mineral-infused oil perfectly complements your dry brushing and gua sha routine by delivering essential nutrients directly to your tissues.

Ingredients:
- 1/4 cup carrier oil (jojoba or sweet almond work beautifully)
- 1 tablespoon pink salt, finely ground
- 5 drops of grapefruit essential oil (lymph stimulator)
- 3 drops cypress essential oil (circulation booster)

- Small glass bottle for storage

Instructions:
1. Warm the carrier oil slightly (not hot)
2. Add pink salt and stir until partially dissolved
3. Add essential oils and mix thoroughly
4. Store in a sealed glass container
5. Shake well before each use

How to Use: Apply a small amount after dry brushing and before gua sha to maximize mineral penetration and enhance lymphatic flow.

3-Minute Lymphatic Reset Routine

This powerful sequence moves stagnant lymph and delivers minerals exactly where your body needs them most.

Step 1: Dry Brushing Sequence
1. Always brush toward your heart using firm but comfortable pressure
2. Start at your feet and work upward in long, sweeping motions
3. Focus extra attention on thighs and upper arms
4. Spend 60-90 seconds covering your entire body

Step 2: Apply Pink Salt Mineral Oil
1. Focus on cellulite-prone areas and lymph-rich zones
2. Use gentle circular motions to enhance absorption

Step 3: Facial Gua Sha Technique
1. Apply the oil to your face and neck
2. Hold the gua sha tool flat against skin at a 45° angle
3. Start at the center of the face and stroke outward and upward
4. Move from jawline to ears, from chin to temples
5. Stroke from the collarbone up the neck to drain the facial fluid

For maximum lymphatic benefits, perform this routine in the morning before your shower and Pink Salt Trick drink. For optimal results, repeat 3 to 4 times weekly.

When your lymphatic system flows freely, everything changes. Metabolism revs up, skin clarifies, and those stubborn fat deposits finally begin to budge! This powerful pink salt ritual delivers results you can see and feel immediately!

Bringing it Together

Your morning Pink Salt Trick drink is a complete game-changer on its own (hello, metabolism!), layering these additional pink salt rituals creates a synergy that transforms your entire body ecosystem.

Think of it like this: your daily pink salt elixir works from the inside out, flooding your cells with trace minerals that kickstart your fat-burning furnace. But when you add these beauty and wellness applications, you're creating a 360-degree approach that leaves no stone unturned in your transformation journey!

Each additional pink salt ritual you incorporate targets a different body system. The result? A complete body reset that addresses weight loss from multiple angles simultaneously.

Pairing your Pink Salt Trick with even gentle exercise creates a metabolic perfect storm. The minerals in pink salt support proper muscle function, hydration, and recovery, which means your workouts become dramatically more effective. Even something as simple as a 20-minute walk after your morning elixir can double your results.

As for nutrition, pink salt minerals help balance your body's pH and electrolytes, creating the optimal environment for digestion and nutrient absorption. This means you'll naturally start craving foods that support your body rather than fighting constant sugar and carb cravings that sabotage your efforts.

But here's what I really want you to understand: This journey isn't just about watching the scale drop (though it probably will). True transformation shows up in countless ways that matter so much more:

- Waking up with energy instead of reaching for caffeine just to function.
- Noticing your favorite jeans sliding on easily without the dreaded jump-and-wiggle.
- Seeing muscle definition appear in places that were once soft and puffy.
- Glowing skin that needs less makeup to look amazing.
- Standing taller with confidence that radiates from the inside out.
- Feeling strong and capable in your daily activities.
- Watching inflammation fade as rings slip on more easily and face puffiness disappears.

These non-scale victories often appear before significant weight drops, and they're powerful indicators that your body is healing and transforming at the cellular level. This is sustainable change, not another quick fix that leaves you right back where you started!

By embracing the complete Pink Salt Trick, your daily drink, targeted beauty rituals, gentle movement, and mineral-supported nutrition, you're not just losing weight. You're rewiring your body's fundamental operating system to work optimally again. You deserve the incredible body healthy body that awaits you!

Conclusion

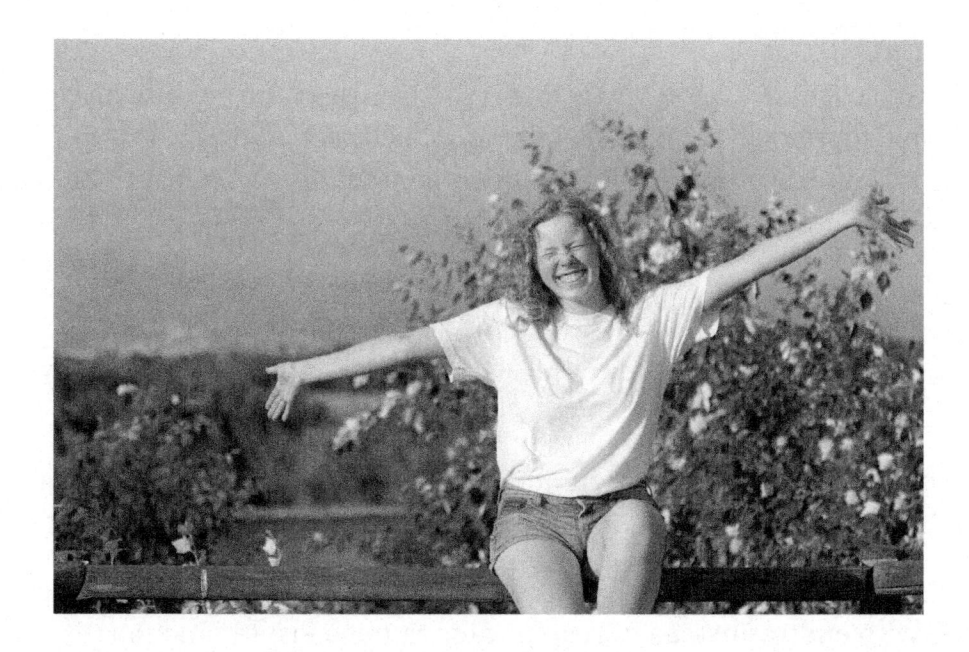

WELL, LOOK AT YOU! From the moment you picked up this book, something inside you whispered, "This time will be different." And guess what? You were absolutely right! By taking a deeper dive into the Pink Salt Trick, you've finally found what your body has been desperately craving all along. Not another punishing diet or expensive supplement, but the simple, mineral-rich solution that nature perfectly designed for your incredible body.

Let's take a moment to celebrate how far you've come on this journey. Remember how you felt before? Those 3 PM energy crashes that sent you diving for coffee and cookies. The frustrating bloat that made your favorite jeans feel like torture devices by dinner. The hormonal rollercoaster that left you wondering if your body was secretly plotting against you. Those days are behind you now!

Instead, you've experienced the almost magical transformation that happens when your cells finally receive the minerals they've been starving for. Your metabolism has awakened from its stubborn slumber. Your hormones have found their natural rhythm again. Your gut is finally processing food the way it was designed to. And the results? They speak for themselves!

Your Pink Salt journey started with something so beautifully simple: a morning glass of mineral-rich drink that takes literally seconds to prepare. No complicated recipes. No expensive ingredients. No time-consuming rituals. Just pure, pink crystalline magic dissolved in water that floods your system with exactly what it needs to thrive. How revolutionary that something so simple could be so powerful!

But you didn't stop there! You've discovered how to incorporate this mineral miracle into every aspect of your life, from beauty routines that make expensive spa treatments look laughable to quick detox practices that flush out toxins and reveal the gorgeous woman who was hiding underneath all along. You've learned how to pair pink salt with movement to create the perfect metabolism-boosting combination. You've seen how these minerals transform not just your weight, but your entire well-being from the inside out.

The best part? This isn't another "lose-weight-quick" scheme that leaves you right back where you started. The Pink Salt Trick works because it addresses the root cause of why your body was struggling in the first place: mineral deficiency that was sabotaging your every effort. By restoring these essential building blocks, you've created lasting change at the cellular level. This is truly a sustainable transformation.

While the weight loss industry wants you to drop hundreds on their latest products, you've discovered that one of the most powerful health tools on the planet costs pennies per day. You don't need fancy equipment, expensive supplements, or complicated meal plans. You just need this humble pink crystal that connects you to ancient wisdom while delivering thoroughly modern results.

Your Experience Could Help Thousands of Women!

You've experienced the Pink Salt Trick transformation firsthand! Those incredible results weren't just in your imagination. Now, imagine another woman, scrolling through Amazon late at night, desperately seeking something that actually works after years of frustration. Your review could be the sign she needs to finally try something different!

It takes just 60 seconds to share your experience, but those few moments could literally change someone's life. Whether you've lost stubborn pounds, regained your energy, or simply feel like yourself again, your honest feedback creates a ripple effect of transformation!

Amazon reviews make all the difference in helping other women discover this mineral magic. Would you take a minute to share your Pink Salt journey? Just scan the QR code below to write your review.

As you close this book, I want you to recognize something profound: you didn't just lose weight. You reclaimed your power. You remembered that your body isn't broken; it was just missing critical nutrients. You've proven to yourself that transformation doesn't have to be complicated or painful. And most importantly, you've created a foundation for lifelong well-being that will continue to serve you for years to come.

The Pink Salt Trick fits seamlessly into any lifestyle because it works with your body, not against it. Whether you're a busy mom juggling a million responsibilities, a career woman with barely a minute to breathe, or someone who's tried literally everything else with disappointing results, this approach meets you exactly where you are. No judgment, no impossible standards, just simple solutions that actually work.

So what happens now? You keep going, beautiful! Continue your morning ritual. Incorporate those pink salt beauty practices that make you feel amazing. Listen to your newly balanced body when it tells you what it needs. Celebrate every non-scale victory along the way. And remember that this journey isn't about achieving some "perfect" end result. It's about living every day in a body that feels energized, capable, and alive!

Your Pink Salt Revolution has only just begun. Here's to your healthiest, happiest, most vibrant life ahead!

References

Aparna M.D., K. (2025). *Redirecting*. Google.com. https://oneworldayurveda.com/blog/amazing-benefits-himalayan-salt-pink-salt/

Ava. (2024, May). *Himalayan pink salt benefits for weight loss*. ERSALY. https://www.ersaly.com/himalayan-pink-salt-benefits-for-weight-loss/

Breaking Down the Health Benefits of Himalayan Pink Salt. (2021, November 16). Sea Salt Superstore. https://www.seasaltsuperstore.com/blogs/what-is-salt/health-benefits-himalayan-pink-salt

Contributors, W. E. (2022, December 5). *Himalayan Salt: Is It Good for You?* WebMD. https://www.webmd.com/diet/himalayan-salt-good-for-you

Does Pink Himalayan Salt Really Help You Lose Weight? The Science Behind the Trend – healthy blog. (2025, May 5). Virginia.edu. https://sites.uvacreate.virginia.edu/health/does-pink-himalayan-salt-really-help-you-lose-weight-the-science-behind-the-trend/

Hall, H. (2017, January 31). *Pink Himalayan Sea Salt: An Update | Science-Based Medicine*. Sciencebasedmedicine.org. https://sciencebasedmedicine.org/pink-himalayan-sea-salt-an-update/

Hall, K. D., & Kahan, S. (2018). Maintenance of lost weight and long-term management of obesity. *Medical Clinics of North America*, *102*(1), 183–197. Ncbi. https://doi.org/10.1016/j.mcna.2017.08.012

Hopkins Medicine. (2025). *Maintaining Weight Loss*. Www.hopkinsmedicine.org. https://www.hopkinsmedicine.org/health/wellness-and-prevention/maintaining-weight-loss

Horstman, E. (2023, February 6). *A Health Coach Shares Her Own Energizing Morning Routine—And It's So Achievable*. Camille Styles. https://camillestyles.com/wellness/holistic-rituals/

Leonard, J. (2018, July 30). *Pink Himalayan salt: Does it have any health benefits?* Www.medicalnewstoday.com. https://www.medicalnewstoday.com/articles/315081

M. Zelman, K. (2024, October 15). *Health Benefits of Sole Water*. WebMD. https://www.webmd.com/diet/health-benefits-sole-water

Radhakrishnan, R. (2021, October 12). *What Are the Benefits of Himalayan Salt?* MedicineNet. https://www.medicinenet.com/what_are_the_benefits_of_himalayan_salt/article.htm

Richards, L. (2023, May 4). *Meditation for weight loss: Research and more*. Www.medicalnewstoday.com. https://www.medicalnewstoday.com/articles/meditation-for-weight-loss

Sareen, S. (2020, August 11). *Medicinal uses of Himalayan pink salt - Rangdaar Online*. Rangdaar.com. https://www.rangdaar.com/blog/medicinal-uses-of-himalayan-pink-salt/

Singh, M.D, R. (2025). *Redirecting*. Google.com. https://pharmeasy.in/blog/ayurveda-uses-benefits-precautions-of-pink-himalayan-salt/

Slimjaro. (2025, April 19). *Pink Salt Trick for Weight Loss: Proven Recipe to Burn Fat Inside Slimjaro Ingredients*. GlobeNewswire News Room; Slimjaro. https://www.globenewswire.com/news-release/2025/04/19/3064398/0/en/Pink-Salt-Trick-for-Weight-Loss-Proven-Recipe-to-Burn-Fat-Inside-Slimjaro-Ingredients.html

Wing, R. R., & Phelan, S. (2005). Long-term weight loss maintenance. *The American Journal of Clinical Nutrition*, *82*(1), 222S225S. https://doi.org/10.1093/ajcn/82.1.222s

Image References

All images supplied by FreePik. www.freepik.com

Printed in Dunstable, United Kingdom